Early Detection of Prostate Cancer

Editors

STACY LOEB
MATTHEW R. COOPERBERG

UROLOGIC CLINICS
OF NORTH AMERICA

www.urologic.theclinics.com

Consulting Editor
SAMIR S. TANEJA

May 2014 • Volume 41 • Number 2

ELSEVIER

1600 John F. Kennedy Boulevard • Suite 1800 • Philadelphia, Pennsylvania, 19103-2899

http://www.theclinics.com

UROLOGIC CLINICS OF NORTH AMERICA Volume 41, Number 2
May 2014 ISSN 0094-0143, ISBN-13: 978-0-323-29725-7

Editor: Kerry Holland
Developmental Editor: Susan Showalter

Urologic Clinics of North America (ISSN 0094-0143) is published quarterly by Elsevier Inc., 360 Park Avenue South, New York, NY 10010-1710. Months of issue are February, May, August, and November. Business and Editorial Offices: 1600 John F. Kennedy Blvd., Suite 1800, Philadelphia, PA 19103-2899. Periodicals postage paid at New York, NY and additional mailing offices. Subscription prices are $355.00 per year (US individuals), $602.00 per year (US institutions), $415.00 per year (Canadian individuals), $752.00 per year (Canadian institutions), $515.00 per year (foreign individuals), and $752.00 per year (foreign institutions). Foreign air speed delivery is included in all *Clinics* subscription prices. All prices are subject to change without notice. **POSTMASTER:** Send address changes to *Urologic Clinics of North America*, Elsevier Health Sciences Division, Subscription Customer Service, 3251 Riverport Lane, Maryland Heights, MO 63043. Customer Service: 1-800-654-2452 (US). From outside the United States, call 1-314-447-8871. Fax: 1-314-447-8029. E-mail: JournalsCustomerServiceusa@elsevier.com (for print support) and JournalsOnlineSupport-usa@elsevier.com (for online support).

Reprints. For copies of 100 or more, of articles in this publication, please contact the Commercial Reprints Department, Elsevier Inc., 360 Park Avenue South, New York, New York 10010-1710. Tel.: 212-633-3874; Fax: 212-633-3820; E-mail: reprints@elsevier.com.

Urologic Clinics of North America is covered in MEDLINE/PubMed (*Index Medicus*), *Excerpta Medica, Current Contents/ Clinical Medicine, Science Citation Index,* and *ISI/BIOMED.*

PROGRAM OBJECTIVE

The goal of Urologic Clinics of North America is to keep practicing urologists and urology residents up to date with current clinical practice in urology by providing timely articles reviewing the state of the art in patient care.

TARGET AUDIENCE

Practicing urologists, urology residents and other health care professionals practicing in the discipline of urology.

LEARNING OBJECTIVES

Upon completion of this activity, participants will be able to:
1. Review technique and complications of prostate biopsy.
2. Discuss the epidemiology and clinical implications of genetic variation in prostate cancer.
3. Explain the management of a rising PSA after negative prostate biopsy.

ACCREDITATION

The Elsevier Office of Continuing Medical Education (EOCME) is accredited by the Accreditation Council for Continuing Medical Education (ACCME) to provide continuing medical education for physicians.

The EOCME designates this enduring material for a maximum of 15 *AMA PRA Category 1 Credit*(s)™. Physicians should claim only the credit commensurate with the extent of their participation in the activity.

All other health care professionals requesting continuing education credit for this enduring material will be issued a certificate of participation.

DISCLOSURE OF CONFLICTS OF INTEREST

The EOCME assesses conflict of interest with its instructors, faculty, planners, and other individuals who are in a position to control the content of CME activities. All relevant conflicts of interest that are identified are thoroughly vetted by EOCME for fair balance, scientific objectivity, and patient care recommendations. EOCME is committed to providing its learners with CME activities that promote improvements or quality in healthcare and not a specific proprietary business or a commercial interest.

The planning committee, staff, authors and editors listed below have identified no financial relationships or relationships to products or devices they or their spouse/life partner have with commercial interest related to the content of this CME activity:

David M. Berman, MD, PhD; Marc A. Bjurlin, DO; Richard J. Bryant, FRCSEd(Urol), PhD; Peter R. Carroll, MD, MPH; Edward K. Chang, BS; Jonathan I. Epstein, MD; Ruth D. Etzioni, PhD; Kirsten L. Greene, MD, MS; Brian T. Helfand, MD, PhD; Kerry Holland; Brynne Hunter; Samuel D. Kaffenberger, MD; Sara J. Knight, PhD; Indu Kumari; Leonard S. Marks, MD; Selma Masic, MD; Jill McNair; Hao Nguyen, MD; Lindsay Parnell; David F. Penson, MD, MPH; Sanoj Punnen, MD, MS; Monique J. Roobol, PhD, MSc; Katsuto Shinohara, MD; Samuel K. Stephenson, MS; James S. Wysock, MD, MSCI.

The planning committee, staff, authors and editors listed below have identified financial relationships or relationships to products or devices they or their spouse/life partner have with commercial interest related to the content of this CME activity:

William J. Catalona, MD is a consultant/advisor for Beckman Coulter, deCode Genetics, OHMX and Nanosphere; has research grants from Beckman Coulter, deCode Genetics, OHMX and Nanosphere; is on speakers bureau for Beckman Coulter; and has royalties/patents from OHMX.

Matthew R. Cooperberg, MD, MPH is a consultant/advisor for Genomic Health, Myriad Genetics, GenomeDX, Astellas, Dendreon, Abbott Labs and Janssen.

Hans Lilja, MD, PhD has stock ownership and royalties/patents with Arctic Partners.

Stacy Loeb, MD, MSCI is consultant/advisor at Sanofi; received honorarium for speaking.

Samir S. Taneja, MD is a consultant/advisor for Eigen, GTX, Bayer, Healthtronics and Hitachi.

Ian M. Thompson, MD is a consultant/advisor for Exosphere Diagnostics and has grants from the National Cancer Institute.

UNAPPROVED/OFF-LABEL USE DISCLOSURE

The EOCME requires CME faculty to disclose to the participants:
1. When products or procedures being discussed are off-label, unlabelled, experimental, and/or investigational (not US Food and Drug Administration (FDA) approved); and
2. Any limitations on the information presented, such as data that are preliminary or that represent ongoing research, interim analyses, and/or unsupported opinions. Faculty may discuss information about pharmaceutical agents that is outside of FDA-approved labelling. This information is intended solely for CME and is not intended to promote off-label use of these medications. If you have any questions, contact the medical affairs department of the manufacturer for the most recent prescribing information.

TO ENROLL

To enroll in the *Urologic Clinics of North America* Continuing Medical Education program, call customer service at 1-800-654-2452 or sign up online at http://www.theclinics.com/home/cme. The CME program is available to subscribers for an additional annual fee of $270 USD.

METHOD OF PARTICIPATION

In order to claim credit, participants must complete the following:

1. Complete enrolment as indicated above.
2. Read the activity.
3. Complete the CME Test and Evaluation. Participants must achieve a score of 70% on the test. All CME Tests and Evaluations must be completed online.

CME INQUIRIES/SPECIAL NEEDS

For all CME inquiries or special needs, please contact elsevierCME@elsevier.com.

Contributors

CONSULTING EDITOR

SAMIR S. TANEJA, MD
The James M. Neissa and Janet Riha Neissa
Professor of Urologic Oncology, Professor of
Urology and Radiology, Director, Division of
Urologic Oncology, Department of Urology,
Co-Director, Smilow Comprehensive Prostate
Cancer Center, New York University Langone
Medical Center, New York, New York

EDITORS

STACY LOEB, MD, MSc
Assistant Professor of Urology and Population
Health, New York University and Manhattan
Veterans Affairs Medical Center, New York,
New York

MATTHEW R. COOPERBERG, MD, MPH
Associate Professor, Departments of Urology
and Epidemiology and Biostatistics, Helen
Diller Family Chair in Urology, University of
California, San Francisco, California

AUTHORS

DAVID M. BERMAN, MD, PhD
Department of Pathology and Molecular
Medicine, Queen's Cancer Research Institute,
Queen's University, Kingston, Ontario,
Canada

MARC A. BJURLIN, DO
Fellow, Division of Urologic Oncology,
Department of Urology, New York University
Langone Medical Center, New York, New York

**RICHARD J. BRYANT, BMedSci(Hons),
MBChB(Hons), FRCSEd(Urol), PhD**
Clinical Lecturer in Urology, Nuffield
Department of Surgical Sciences, John
Radcliffe Hospital, University of Oxford,
Headley Way, Headington, Oxford,
United Kingdom

PETER R. CARROLL, MD, MPH
Department of Urology, UCSF Helen Diller
Family Comprehensive Cancer Center,
University of California, San Francisco,
San Francisco, California

WILLIAM J. CATALONA, MD
Professor of Urology, Department of Urology,
Feinberg School of Medicine, Northwestern
University, Chicago, Illinois

EDWARD K. CHANG, BS
Research Associate, Department of Urology,
Geffen School of Medicine at UCLA,
Los Angeles, California

JONATHAN I. EPSTEIN, MD
Departments of Pathology, Oncology, and
Urology, The Johns Hopkins Medical
Institutions, Baltimore, Maryland

RUTH D. ETZIONI, PhD
Division of Public Health Sciences, Fred
Hutchinson Cancer Research Center, Seattle,
Washington

KIRSTEN L. GREENE, MD, MS
Department of Urology, UCSF Helen Diller
Family Comprehensive Cancer Center,
University of California, San Francisco,
San Francisco, California

BRIAN T. HELFAND, MD, PhD
Assistant Professor of Urology, Department of Surgery, NorthShore University HealthSystem, University of Chicago Pritzker School of Medicine, Evanston, Illinois

SAMUEL D. KAFFENBERGER, MD
Chief Resident, Department of Urologic Surgery, Vanderbilt University, Nashville, Tennessee

SARA J. KNIGHT, PhD
Deputy Director, Health Services Research and Development Service, Office of Research and Development, Veterans Health Administration, Washington, DC; Associate Professor, Departments of Psychiatry and Urology, University of California San Francisco, San Francisco, California

HANS LILJA, MD, PhD
Professor of Clinical Biochemistry, Nuffield Department of Surgical Sciences, John Radcliffe Hospital, University of Oxford, Headley Way, Headington, Oxford, United Kingdom; Member, Attending Clinical Chemist, Departments of Laboratory Medicine, Surgery (Urology), and Medicine (GU-Oncology), Memorial Sloan-Kettering Cancer Center, New York, New York

LEONARD S. MARKS, MD
Professor of Urology, Department of Urology, Geffen School of Medicine at UCLA, Los Angeles, California

SELMA MASIC, MD
Resident, Department of Urology, University of California, San Francisco, San Francisco, California

HAO NGUYEN, MD
Fellow in Urological Oncology, Department of Urology, University of California, San Francisco, San Francisco, California

DAVID F. PENSON, MD, MPH
Staff Physician, VA Tennessee Valley Geriatric Research, Education, and Clinical Center

(GRECC); Hamilton and Howd Chair in Urologic Oncology, Director, Center for Surgical Quality and Outcomes Research, Professor of Urologic Surgery and Medicine, Vanderbilt University, Nashville, Tennessee

SANOJ PUNNEN, MD, MS
Department of Urology, UCSF Helen Diller Family Comprehensive Cancer Center, University of California, San Francisco, San Francisco, California

MONIQUE J. ROOBOL, PhD, MSc
Associate Professor, Department of Urology, Erasmus University Medical Center, Rotterdam, The Netherlands

KATSUTO SHINOHARA, MD
Helen Diller Family Chair in Clinical Urology, Professor, Department of Urology, University of California, San Francisco, San Francisco, California

SAMUEL K. STEPHENSON, MS
Medical Student, Department of Urology, Geffen School of Medicine at UCLA, Los Angeles, California

SAMIR S. TANEJA, MD
The James M. Neissa and Janet Riha Neissa Professor of Urologic Oncology, Professor of Urology and Radiology, Director, Division of Urologic Oncology, Department of Urology, Co-Director, Smilow Comprehensive Prostate Cancer Center, New York University Langone Medical Center, New York, New York

IAN M. THOMPSON, MD
The Cancer Therapy and Research Center, University of Texas Health Science Center at San Antonio, San Antonio, Texas

JAMES S. WYSOCK, MD, MSCI
Fellow, Division of Urologic Oncology, Department of Urology, New York University Langone Medical Center, New York, New York

Contents

Publication of apparently conflicting results from 2 large trials of prostate cancer screening has intensified the debate about prostate-specific antigen (PSA) testing and has led to a recommendation against screening from the US Preventive Services Task Force. This article reviews the trials and discusses the limitations of their empirical results in informing public health policy. In particular, the authors explain why harm-benefit trade-offs based on empirical results may not accurately reflect the trade-offs expected under long-term population screening. This information should be useful to clinicians in understanding the implications of these studies regarding the value of PSA screening.

Although observational studies and simulation models have shed some interesting light on many of the uncertainties surrounding prostate cancer screening, well-done clinical trials provide the best evidence on screening among the extremes of age, the most appropriate interval to screen, and the best complement of tests to use. Enthusiasm for screening is temporized by the acknowledgment that overdetection leads to frequent overtreatment despite evidence supporting the safety of active surveillance in many men with low-risk disease.

The estimated population of the world in 2008 was 6.75 billion people, increasing by around 79 million people each year. The world population is aging. In 1970, the world median age was 22 years; it is projected to reach 38 years by 2050. The number of people in the world aged 60 years and older is expected to almost triple to 2 billion by 2050. Because cancer, especially prostate cancer, is predominantly a disease of the elderly, increases in the number of older people will lead to more cases of cancer, even if current incidence rates remain the same.

The controversial recent recommendation by the United States Preventive Services Task Force (USPSTF) against prostate-specific antigen (PSA) screening for early-stage prostate cancer has caused much debate. Whereas USPSTF recommendations against routine screening mammography in younger women resulted in fierce public outcry and eventual alteration in the language of the recommendation, the same public and political response has not been seen with PSA screening for prostate cancer. It is of paramount importance to ensure improved efficiency and transparency of the USPSTF recommendation process, and resolution of concerns with the current USPSTF recommendation against PSA screening for all ages.

Decision Making and Prostate Cancer Screening   257

Sara J. Knight

This article presents an overview of the challenges that men encounter in making decisions about prostate cancer screening, including complex affective and cognitive factors and controversies in the interpretation of the evidence on prostate cancer screening. Shared decision making involving patient decision aids are discussed as approaches that can be used to improve the quality of prostate cancer screening decisions, including a close alignment between a man's values, goals, and preferences and his choice about screening.

Emerging PSA-Based Tests to Improve Screening   267

Richard J. Bryant and Hans Lilja

This article updates advances in prostate cancer screening based on prostate-specific antigen, its derivatives, and human kallikrein markers. Many men are diagnosed with indolent disease not requiring treatment. Although there is evidence of a survival benefit from screening, the numbers needed to screen and treat remain high. There is risk of exposing men to the side effects of treatment for nonthreatening disease. A screening test is needed with sufficiently good performance characteristics to detect disease at an early stage so treatment may be offered with curative intent, while reducing the number of negative or unnecessary biopsies.

The Epidemiology and Clinical Implications of Genetic Variation in Prostate Cancer   277

Brian T. Helfand and William J. Catalona

There is strong evidence of a genetic predisposition to prostate cancer. Recent advances in genetic sequencing technologies have permitted significant advances in the field. This article reviews the genetic basis underlying prostate cancer, and highlights the epidemiology and potential clinical usefulness of both rare and common genetic variations. In addition, recent findings related to the understanding of prostate cancer genetics are discussed.

Optimization of Prostate Biopsy: Review of Technique and Complications   299

Marc A. Bjurlin, James S. Wysock, and Samir S. Taneja

A 12-core systematic biopsy that incorporates apical and far-lateral cores in the template distribution allows maximal cancer detection and avoidance of a repeat biopsy while minimizing the detection of insignificant prostate cancers. Magnetic resonance imaging–guided prostate biopsy has an evolving role in both initial and repeat prostate biopsy strategies, potentially improving sampling efficiency, increasing the detection of clinically significant cancers, and reducing the detection of insignificant cancers. Hematuria, hematospermia, and rectal bleeding are common complications of prostate needle biopsy, but are generally self-limiting and well tolerated. All men should receive antimicrobial prophylaxis before biopsy.

Screening and Detection Advances in Magnetic Resonance Image–Guided Prostate Biopsy

Samuel K. Stephenson, Edward K. Chang, and Leonard S. Marks

Multiparametric magnetic resonance imaging (MRI) has provided a method for visualizing prostate cancer. MRI-ultrasonography fusion allows prostate biopsy to be performed quickly, on an outpatient basis, using the transrectal technique. Targeted biopsies are more sensitive for detection of prostate cancer than nontargeted, systematic biopsies and detect more significant prostate cancers and fewer insignificant cancers than conventional biopsies. A negative MRI scan should not defer biopsy. Two groups who will especially benefit from targeted prostate biopsy are men with low-risk lesions in active surveillance and men with increased prostate-specific antigen levels and previous negative conventional biopsies.

Management of an Increasing Prostate-Specific Antigen Level After Negative Prostate Biopsy

Katsuto Shinohara, Hao Nguyen, and Selma Masic

Patients who have a previously negative biopsy in the setting of clinical suspicion of prostate cancer still have a high risk of harboring significant undiagnosed disease. Various markers such as prostate-specific antigen (PSA) velocity, PSA density, PCA3, and newer markers may aid in repeat biopsy selection. Repeating the same biopsy procedure in such patients does not yield high cancer detection rates. More anteriorly directed transrectal or transperineal biopsies are indicated. Multiparametric magnetic resonance imaging can detect abnormal areas, and lesion-targeted biopsies can improve the cancer detection rate.

When is Prostate Cancer Really Cancer?

David M. Berman and Jonathan I. Epstein

Several investigators have challenged the idea that low-grade cancers are a cause for concern, suggesting that the term cancer should not be applied to these tumors. This article reviews the defining features of cancer, and the diagnostic and prognostic classification systems currently used for prostate cancer. Logical, morphologic, and molecular evidence is presented to show that low-grade prostate cancers are correctly classified as cancer. The authors suggest, however, that 6 out of 10 on an aggressiveness scale is inappropriate for indolent cancer, and that a proposed reinterpretation of Gleason grading categories is a more logical way to address overtreatment.

Index

UROLOGIC CLINICS OF NORTH AMERICA

Foreword
Early Detection of Prostate Cancer

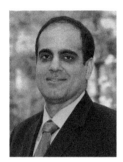

Samir S. Taneja, MD
Consulting Editor

During the period of my career in Urology, we have come full circle in the arena of prostate cancer. As a student in the 1980s, I learned to diagnose prostate cancer by digital rectal exam and observation of clinical symptoms. I observed men dying from metastatic disease, requiring channel TURP for retention, and on rare occasion, watched as the residents gathered around to absorb the occasional radical prostatectomy.

In the 1990s, during my residency training and early practice, I watched an enthusiastic groundswell behind the introduction of PSA, the transition from digital-guided biopsy to ultrasound-guided biopsy, and the description and refinement of the nerve-sparing radical prostatectomy. We strived to diagnose disease earlier and earlier because we believed we were advancing the disease further and further away from the horrible oncologic outcomes of the 1970s and 1980s.

In the 2000s, the focus turned to the side effects of therapy and its impact on quality of life, and slowly we began to question whether earlier diagnosis and treatment were really beneficial to our patients. Studies were completed that demonstrated modest reductions in mortality, but a substantial cost, measured in dollars and patient investment, associated with the process of diagnosing and curing the disease.

In part, our ability to be so critical of our own practice stemmed from the fact that we rarely now see men coming to us debilitated from the disease. With the memory of spinal cord compressions, bone pain, and surgical orchiectomy so far behind them, our colleagues from other specialties began to treat the disease as an innocuous entity.

As we entered the current decade, I believe we come in with tremendous confusion about how to approach prostate cancer. The medical establishment would advise we don't look for the disease unless the patient is symptomatic. In this way, I am well trained. Having experienced the 1980s, I am very capable of recognizing the pain of advanced disease and managing symptoms without hope of cure. I think, we are not eager, as urologists, to return to that time.

We remain mindful that the disease continues to remain a killer of American men and has the potential to grow in its ability to kill if left unattended. We also recognize that the current one-size-fits-all paradigm of prostate cancer diagnosis followed by radical treatment is unacceptable because not every prostate cancer will kill, and because the secondary consequences of treatment are substantial. This approach is not sustainable. In my view, the decisions we make about prostate cancer detection in the near future are perhaps the most critical in determining the eventual fate of our patients, and of urology practice in general.

The ability to successfully treat patients with cancer as individuals, and to prescribe therapies of true benefit, has several a priori requisites. First, one must be able to contextualize the disease within the setting of an individual host. Learning to assess comorbidities and predict longevity is only part of this. The patient's expectations and pre-existing urologic quality of life

Urol Clin N Am 41 (2014) xi–xii
http://dx.doi.org/10.1016/j.ucl.2014.03.002
0094-0143/14/$ – see front matter © 2014 Published by Elsevier Inc.

must be determined. Second, one must be able risk-stratify the disease and make effort to determine its lethality and its speed. In recent years, several methods of tumor assessment have emerged ranging from predictive biomarkers to noninvasive imaging to genetic assessment of tumor tissue. Finally, one must have a menu of efficacious treatment options that can be tailored to the patient and the tumor. In doing so, side effects can be accepted when necessary, but not imposed on all.

In this most important issue of *Urologic Clinics*, two of the most thoughtful opinion leaders in the field of prostate cancer, Drs Stacy Loeb and Matthew Cooperberg, have constructed a comprehensive overview of the current state of prostate cancer screening, detection, and molecular risk stratification. In doing so, they have offered insight into the tools available to construct future, individualized, approaches to the disease. Our guest editors have constructed a broad table of contents to include articles on the most relevant aspects of the prostate cancer controversy from some of our community's most respected colleagues. The issue offers the reader a chance to be well versed in those approaches to disease detection and risk stratification most likely to be utilized in redefining the current approach to prostate cancer.

I am deeply indebted to Drs Loeb and Cooperberg for taking on this arduous task, and to each of the contributors for a job extremely well done. I sincerely hope that the readers will use this issue as a means of leaping forward into the next decade of prostate cancer management.

Samir S. Taneja, MD
Division of Urologic Oncology
Smilow Comprehensive Prostate Cancer Center
Department of Urology
NYU Langone Medical Center
150 East 32nd Street, Suite 200
New York, NY 10016, USA

E-mail address:
samir.taneja@nyumc.org

Preface
Early Detection of Prostate Cancer

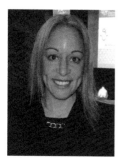
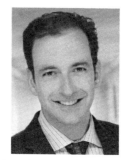

Stacy Loeb, MD, MSc   Matthew R. Cooperberg, MD, MPH

Editors

Although prostate cancer remains the second leading cause of cancer death among men in the United States, in the era of prostate-specific antigen (PSA)-based early-detection efforts, age-adjusted prostate cancer mortality rates in this country have fallen nearly 50%. Despite this favorable epidemiological trend, prostate cancer early detection remains intensely controversial, due in part to highly prevalent overtreatment of low-risk, indolent tumors and to widespread misconceptions regarding the existing evidence supporting early-detection efforts.

As guest editors of this issue of *Urologic Clinics*, it was our goal to provide readers a timely summary of some of the key controversies in prostate cancer early detection and how these issues might be resolved in the future. The first set of articles in this issue explores in detail the evidence for and against the mortality benefits associated with PSA testing, the evolving incorporation of this evidence into early-detection guidelines and shared decision-making models in the Unites States and abroad, and the political aspects of the PSA debate particularly as they relate to the US Preventive Services Task Force recommendation to end all PSA-based early-detection efforts.

In addition, there are many new biomarkers in the pipeline that hold the potential to improve early-detection efforts. These range from newly discovered germline genetic variants to PSA isoforms and related molecules, to better imaging modalities. This issue also reviews some of the most recent developments in this area.

Finally, other articles in this issue highlight technical aspects of ultrasound-guided and MRI-guided prostate biopsy, the management of elevated PSA after a negative biopsy, and a perspective on the emerging question of whether low-grade prostate cancer should in fact be called "cancer."

The authors of these articles include some of the best thought leaders in the world on these questions. We are thankful to them for their contributions to this issue and are extremely appreciative of the significant amount of time and insight that they have provided on this critically important topic. We hope and expect these articles will be of great interest to a diverse readership.

Stacy Loeb, MD, MSc
New York University and
Manhattan Veterans Affairs Medical Center
550 1st Avenue, VZ30 (6th Floor, #612)
New York, NY 10016, USA

Matthew R. Cooperberg, MD, MPH
Departments of Urology and
Epidemiology and Biostatistics
Helen Diller Family Chair in Urology
University of California, San Francisco
San Francisco, CA, USA

E-mail addresses:
stacyloeb@gmail.com (S. Loeb)
mcooperberg@urology.ucsf.edu (M.R. Cooperberg)

Urol Clin N Am 41 (2014) xiii
http://dx.doi.org/10.1016/j.ucl.2014.03.001
0094-0143/14/$ – see front matter © 2014 Published by Elsevier Inc.

What Do the Screening Trials Really Tell Us and Where Do We Go From Here?

Ruth D. Etzioni, PhD[a],*, Ian M. Thompson, MD[b]

KEYWORDS

- Prostate cancer • Mass screening • Clinical trials • Prostate-specific antigen • Simulation modeling
- Public health policy

KEY POINTS

- Screening trials provide information that is critical for the development of screening policy, but cannot provide all the information needed for developing sound policies for population screening.
- Results from a modeling analysis of the Prostate, Lung, Colon, and Ovarian trial reveals that the empirical finding of no difference in prostate cancer mortality in this study could have easily occurred even if prostate cancer screening had a high degree of efficacy.
- The balance of screening harm with benefit will be materially affected by patient decisions following diagnosis, such as whether the patient selects aggressive curative treatment or active surveillance to reduce the chance of overtreatment.

INTRODUCTION

The prostate screening odyssey has captivated researchers, policymakers, and clinicians since the late 1980s when the prostate-specific antigen (PSA) test was approved by the Food and Drug Administration for monitoring the progression of prostate cancer. The test was rapidly adopted for screening in the United States[1] even as clinical trials to evaluate its efficacy in early detection were just beginning in the United States and Europe.

While the United States and European trials were ongoing, routine PSA screening became the standard of care in the United States, dramatically changing the profile of prostate cancer, and prompting concerns about overdetection and overtreatment of the disease. As rates of death from prostate cancer declined after the inception

of screening, it became clear that policies for prostate cancer screening would have to carefully navigate the harm-benefit trade-offs of PSA testing. The results of the 2 large, randomized screening trials were eagerly awaited for what was hoped would be the final word regarding the lives saved and the price that would have to be paid for any screening benefit.

Five years after the publication of the primary trial results, there remains a vigorous debate about whether and how best to screen for prostate cancer. The randomized trial results were the basis for revised prostate screening recommendations from all of the major policy panels including the US Preventive Services Task Force (USPSTF),[2] the American Cancer Society,[3] and the American Urology Association.[4] Whereas the USPSTF has

Supported by U01 CA157224 (Cancer Intervention and Surveillance Modeling Network from the National Cancer Institute), P30 CA015704-36 (Cancer Center Support Grant from the National Cancer Institute) and U01 CA86402 (from the Early Detection Research Network of the National Cancer Institute).

[a] Division of Public Health Sciences, Fred Hutchinson Cancer Research Center, 1100 Fairview Avenue North, M2-B230, PO Box 19024, Seattle, WA 98109-1024, USA; [b] The Cancer Therapy and Research Center, University of Texas Health Science Center at San Antonio, MC-7845, 7703 Floyd Curl Drive, San Antonio, TX 78229-3900, USA
* Corresponding author.
E-mail address: retzioni@fhcrc.org

Urol Clin N Am 41 (2014) 223–228
http://dx.doi.org/10.1016/j.ucl.2014.01.002
0094-0143/14/$ – see front matter © 2014 Elsevier Inc. All rights reserved.

recommended against PSA screening at all ages, the other panels have generally recommended shared decision making except for men with a limited life expectancy.

This article reexamines the trials and their findings in light of what needs to be known to develop policies for population screening. The authors first review the empiric results from the trials and ask what they inform us about (1) screening benefit, (2) screening harms, particularly overdiagnosis, and (3) the harm-benefit trade-offs of screening. Statistical and modeling analyses that go beyond the trial results are considered, and how these results may modify perceptions of the aforementioned outcomes is discussed. All screening outcomes depend on the screening strategy used, including the screening ages, intervals, and cutoffs for biopsy referral. Varying these parameters can dramatically alter the balance of harm and benefit; unfortunately, the 2 randomized trials are inherently limited in their ability to compare alternative screening strategies. The authors conclude that screening trials in general, and the Prostate, Lung, Colon, and Ovarian (PLCO) trial and European Randomized Study of Screening for Prostate Cancer (ERSPC) in particular, provide information that is critical for the development of screening policy, but cannot provide all the information needed for developing sound policies for population screening.

THE LARGE RANDOMIZED PROSTATE CANCER SCREENING TRIALS

The 2 large screening trials, the United States–based PLCO cancer screening trial[5,6] and the ERSPC,[7,8] have been previously described in detail.

Several measures of screening benefit and harm are presented in the trial reports, and these are briefly reviewed here, as the manner by which harm and benefit are measured will significantly influence the perception of the value of screening. Several definitions are important in understanding screening outcomes. The relative screening benefit is expressed by the (prostate cancer) mortality rate ratio, which is the ratio of the risk of death from prostate cancer in the screened group relative to the control group over the follow-up period. The absolute screening benefit is expressed by the difference between the cumulative incidence of death from prostate cancer in the 2 groups, and may be thought of as an estimate of the lives saved by screening over the follow-up period. Both relative and absolute benefits are time-sensitive and generally increase with follow-up time.[9–11] Overdiagnosis is the detection by

screening of cases that, in the absence of screening, would not have caused morbidity or mortality in the patient's lifetime. Overdiagnosis may be expressed as an absolute number of over-diagnosed cases, as a fraction of the number screened, or as a fraction of screen-detected cases. Depending on how overdiagnosis is estimated, the results may also be highly time-sensitive. Finally, a measure of harm-benefit trade-off that has become fairly standard is the (additional) number needed to detect (NND) to prevent 1 death from prostate cancer, defined as the estimated overdiagnoses divided by the estimated lives saved by screening. The NND has been referred to as the additional number needed to treat to prevent 1 death from prostate cancer but this is not, strictly speaking, accurate, because not all newly diagnosed prostate cancers receive immediate treatment. The concept of the NND, a harm-benefit trade-off measure pertaining specifically to screening that carries the possibility of overdiagnosis, should be distinguished from the similarly named number needed to treat or NNT, which is a concept of benefit most commonly used in analysis of treatment trials.

The PLCO Screening Trial

The PLCO trial randomized 76,693 men to screening or a control group managed according to community standards. Screening-arm participants were given annual PSA tests for 6 years with concomitant digital rectal examinations (DREs) for the first 4 years. Diagnostic follow-up for positive test results was left to participants who were referred to their doctors for PSA higher than 4.0 ng/mL or a suspicious finding on DRE. Approximately 40% of participants referred to biopsy for an abnormal screening test underwent prostate biopsy within 1 year.[12]

By the time the PLCO trial began randomizing participants, PSA screening was widespread.[1] This aspect had a critical impact on the trial and its outcomes. In brief, 45% of participants had had at least 1 PSA before enrollment[6]; moreover, over the course of the trial approximately half of the control-arm participants were screened every year, with 74% of the control group receiving at least 1 screening test during their participation in the trial.[13] By contrast, 95% of the screened group was screened at least once during the course of the trial. The average number of screening tests was 5 in the screened group and 2.7 in the control group.[13] Thus, screening in the control group was approximately half as intensive as that in the screened group.

The empirical results from the PLCO after 11 and 13 years of follow-up clearly show no relative or absolute benefit of PSA screening.[5,6] Not only was there no statistically significant difference in prostate cancer mortality between screened and control groups after 11 and 13 years of follow-up, but the cumulative incidence of deaths from prostate cancer was slightly (but nonsignificantly) higher in the screened group than in the control group (mortality rate ratio 1.09, 95% confidence interval 0.87–13.6).

In its recent recommendation against routine PSA screening, the USPSTF concluded that the benefit of PSA screening ranged from zero to 1 life saved per 1000 men screened at 8 to 10 years, with the zero directly based on the results of the PLCO trial.[2] However, it is clear that the trial did not compare screening with no screening; the trial investigators themselves note in their most recent report that the results pertain to annual versus "opportunistic" screening in the United States.[6] By simulating a replication of the trial many times, the authors have shown that even if screening were to confer a clinically significant reduction in prostate cancer mortality, it is unlikely (only 10%–20% chance) that the trial would have produced a statistically significant benefit.[14] In addition, the authors showed that the finding of zero lives saved (or, more generally, fewer deaths in the control group than in the screened group) could reasonably have occurred in practice given that the numbers of deaths in both groups were considerably lower than expected. Thus, deeper analysis of the PLCO results indicates that the trial cannot be interpreted as a negative study regarding the benefit of PSA screening, despite the empirical results concerning disease-specific deaths in the control and intervention arms. Similarly, meta-analyses drawing on the PLCO results that simply use the empirical trial findings as a data point for comparison with the other trial results are not interpretable.

The PLCO trial does provide a great deal of information regarding the comparison of (approximately) annual with opportunistic (approximately half as intensive) screening in the United States. The trial also provides valuable information regarding the false-positive properties of PSA testing as conducted in the trial; among men with a positive test who underwent biopsy, 35% to 45% had prostate cancer detected.[15] Finally, the trial provides important data about the likelihood of compliance with a referral for prostate biopsy in the United States population; only about 40% of participants underwent biopsy within 1 year after a positive test.[12] However, the empirical results do not inform about the benefits of screening versus no screening, the likelihood of overdiagnosis, or the NND.

The ERSPC Screening Trial

The ERSPC was designed as a single trial to evaluate PSA efficacy in European countries that satisfied pilot-study requirements, and incorporated 60% of participants in a trial that had already been started in one center (Göteborg, Sweden).[16] The trial randomized 182,160 men, with the largest number randomized in Finland and the smallest number in Spain. An age range of 55 to 69 years was designated as the core age group and enrolled across all centers, with some centers also including men aged 70 to 74. Testing took place every 4 years in most centers, but every 2 years in Sweden. The criteria for biopsy referral varied across centers. Most centers used a PSA cutoff of 3 ng/mL, whereas Finland used a cutoff of 4 ng/mL. In contrast to the PLCO trial, there was generally excellent compliance with screening and biopsy referral: on average 86% of participants complied with biopsy recommendations.[8] An analysis of contamination across 5 centers of the ERSPC[17] reveals variable frequencies of opportunistic screening, with annual rates of less than 10% in Finland, the Netherlands, and Spain, and higher rates (20%–30% per year) in Italy and France.

The primary outcome of the ERSPC differs from that of the PLCO: At 11 years of follow-up there was a statistically significant 21% relative reduction in the prostate cancer mortality rate in the intervention group.[8] As 5 men per 1000 in the control group died of prostate cancer during the follow-up period, this relative reduction amounted to 1 life saved per 1000 men screened. After accounting for noncompliance and contamination, the relative mortality reduction increased to 31%.[18] Overdiagnosis was estimated as the excess cases of prostate cancer in the intervention relative to the control group (37 per 1000 men screened). The corresponding estimate of the NND provided by study investigators was 37 at 11 years' follow-up, given by the excess cases in the intervention group divided by the lives saved. **Table 1** summarizes the results of the trial at 11 years of follow-up and also the results of the Swedish,[19] Finnish,[20] and Dutch[21] trials, which have been reported in separate publications.

The ERSPC results have been interpreted as indicating that screening provides at best a very modest benefit at considerable cost in terms of overdiagnosis. Indeed, in the conclusion by USPSTF that the absolute benefit of PSA screening ranged from zero to 1 life saved per 1000 men screened, the upper limit was directly based on the results of the ERSPC after 9 years.

Both the estimate of lives saved (1 per 1000 men screened) and the NND (37 excess cases per life

Table 1
Summary of published reports of primary outcomes from the European Randomized Study of Screening for Prostate Cancer (ERSPC) and the Prostate, Lung, Colon, and Ovarian (PLCO) trial

Study	Age (y)	N	Start Year	Follow-Up (Median Years)	Cum. Inc. of Disease (%) Control	Cum. Inc. of Disease (%) Screened	Cum. Inc. of Prostate Cancer Death (%) Control	Mortality Rate Ratio	Lives Saved Per 1000	NND
ERSPC	55–69	162,388	1991	11	6.00	9.60	0.50	0.79	1.07	37
Rotterdam	55–74	42,376	1993	12.8	6.84	12.75	0.90	0.8	1.8	33
Finland	55–69	80,144	1996	12	6.90	9.00	0.55	0.85	0.83	25
Sweden	50–69	20,000	1994	14	8.20	12.70	0.90	0.56	4	12
PLCO	55–74	76,685	1993	13	9.95	11.09	0.38	1.09	0	Inf

Also presented are reports from the 3 ERSPC sites that published results separately. Cum. Inc. indicates cumulative incidence; the cumulative incidence of disease gives the fraction of participants on each arm diagnosed with prostate cancer during the course of follow-up. The similarity between the incidence on the screened and the control arms of the PLCO trial reflects the contamination by opportunistic screening among control group participants. The cumulative incidence of prostate cancer death gives the fraction of participants on each arm dying of prostate cancer during the course of follow-up. Lives saved represents the difference between these fractions expressed relative to 1000 men enrolled. The mortality rate ratio is the ratio of the risk of prostate cancer death on the screened arm relative to the control arm. The NND (additional number needed to detect) should ideally reflect the ratio of overdiagnoses to deaths prevented; however, studies[11,22] have shown that this is not accurately estimated by limited-term trial data.
    Data from Refs.[6,8,19–21]

saved) have been questioned in further analyses.[22–25] First, when considered against a background mortality that is more reflective of the lifetime risk of death from prostate cancer, the number of lives saved given annual screening of men aged 50 to 69 increases considerably, to 9 per 1000 men screened in Europe[24] and 5 to 6 per 1000 men screened in the United States.[25] Some of the differences between the United States and European estimates of lives saved can likely be attributed to differences in background mortality, screening protocols (the European estimate used a PSA cutoff for biopsy referral of 3 ng/mL and the United States estimate was based on a cutoff of 4 ng/mL), and biopsy compliance rates. It is noteworthy that, when considering these higher estimates of lives saved against the number of overdiagnosed cases in each setting, the NND is dramatically reduced to approximately 5 in both European and United States settings.[24,25] Thus, deeper analysis of the ERSPC reveals a more favorable picture of both benefit and the harm-benefit trade-offs of PSA screening than has generally been inferred from the empirical results.

WHERE DO WE GO FROM HERE?

There is no question that these 2 randomized screening trials provide us with a wealth of information about PSA screening. However, they also present us with a fundamental question: do empirical findings from randomized trials adequately reflect the true harms and benefits of screening tests? Unfortunately, as illustrated in this review, these studies cannot answer this question, and focusing solely on empirical results, even from these very large high-quality trials, can lead to serious misperceptions regarding the value of prostate cancer screening.

With respect to benefit, results from a modeling analysis of the PLCO trial reveals that the empirical finding of no difference in prostate cancer mortality in this study could have easily occurred even if prostate cancer screening had a high degree of efficacy. The empirical result from the ERSPC regarding relative benefit is clinically significant (20%–30% reduction in the risk of death from prostate cancer), but the empirical findings concerning absolute benefit (lives saved) and the NND (harm to benefit ratio) appear to have eclipsed this finding to yield a general perception of modest benefit outweighed by harm. Statistical and modeling studies targeted at quantifying how these outcomes will likely change over longer follow-up (as would be expected with a policy of screening in clinical practice)[11,22–25] reveal that the empirical results do not accurately reflect the lives saved or the NND that would be expected under population screening. Even the reported mortality rate ratio may well underestimate the percent reduction over the longer term[9]; this seems to be the case as longer-term data are released from the ERSPC, showing greater relative mortality reductions with longer follow-up, and an NND of 37 after 11 years compared with an NND of 48 after 9 years.[8]

In conclusion, screening trial results are traditionally regarded as gold-standard evidence, but we must go beyond the empiric findings of the PLCO and the ERSPC to understand what these trials are really telling us. As deeper scrutiny of the trial outcomes using statistical and modeling analyses strongly suggests a clinically significant benefit from screening, a rational public health approach should be to determine optimal implementation of screening to minimize harm while maximizing benefit.

Recent observational and modeling studies provide some direction for a way forward. Vickers and colleagues[26] studied the association between PSA levels at ages 40 to 55 and the long-term risks of metastasis in an unscreened population. Their findings indicate a strong correlation between higher PSA levels at these ages and the risk of future metastatic disease, and prompt a suggestion to use early PSA testing to stratify men to more versus less intensive screening approaches. Gulati and colleagues[25] compared 35 different policies, varying ages to start and stop screening, intervals between screens, and criteria for biopsy referral. Their results suggest that screening less intensively, particularly if PSA levels are low, and referring to biopsy less readily in men older than 70 could substantially reduce overdiagnosis and false-positive tests while preserving more than 70% of the lives saved under annual screening. Heijnsdijk and colleagues[24] compared fewer policies, also noting that less frequent screening (every 4 years) preserves the majority (two-thirds) of lives saved when compared with annual screening. However, the key conclusion of this study concerned the impacts of treatment and its consequences on the quality-adjusted life-years saved by screening. The specific quality weights used by the investigators imply that screening benefit is highly sensitive to quality of life (quality-adjusted life-years saved were projected to be 23% lower than unadjusted life-years). However, as noted by an accompanying editorial,[27] existing data on the distribution of utilities corresponding to key health states are far from adequate. This study therefore highlights the need for, and the challenge of, accurately quantifying harm-benefit trade-offs when developing screening policies.

It is likely that the harms and benefits of screening will be valued differently by different individuals. The balance of harm to benefit will also be materially affected by patient decisions following diagnosis, such as whether the patient selects aggressive curative treatment or active surveillance to reduce the chance of overtreatment. Ultimately, as acknowledged by current screening guidelines from national panels (eg, Refs.[3,28]) that recommend shared decision making, the optimal approach to prostate cancer screening may well depend on the patient.

REFERENCES

1. Mariotto A, Etzioni R, Krapcho M, et al. Reconstructing prostate-specific antigen (PSA) testing patterns among black and white men in the US from Medicare claims and the National Health Interview Survey. Cancer 2007;109(9):1877–86.
2. Moyer VA, on behalf of the USPSTF. Screening for prostate cancer: U.S. preventive services task force recommendation statement. Ann Intern Med 2012; 157(2):120–34.
3. Wolf AM, Wender RC, Etzioni RB, et al. American Cancer Society guideline for the early detection of prostate cancer: update 2010. CA Cancer J Clin 2010;60(2):70–98.
4. Association AU. Early detection of prostate cancer: AUA guideline. 2013. Available at: http://www.aua net.org/education/guidelines/prostate-cancer-detec tion.cfm. Accessed February 10, 2014.
5. Andriole GL, Crawford ED, Grubb RL 3rd, et al. Mortality results from a randomized prostate-cancer screening trial. N Engl J Med 2009;360(13):1310–9.
6. Andriole GL, Crawford ED, Grubb RL 3rd, et al. Prostate cancer screening in the randomized Prostate, Lung, Colorectal, and Ovarian cancer screening trial: mortality results after 13 years of follow-up. J Natl Cancer Inst 2012;104:1–8.
7. Schröder FH, Hugosson J, Roobol MJ, et al. Screening and prostate-cancer mortality in a randomized European study. N Engl J Med 2009; 360(13):1320–8.
8. Schröder FH, Hugosson J, Roobol MJ, et al. Prostate-cancer mortality at 11 years of follow-up. N Engl J Med 2012;366(11):981–90.
9. Hanley JA. Mortality reductions produced by sustained prostate cancer screening have been underestimated. J Med Screen 2010;17(3):147–51.
10. Hanley JA. Measuring mortality reductions in cancer screening trials. Epidemiol Rev 2011;33(1):36–45.
11. Gulati R, Mariotto AB, Chen S, et al. Long-term projections of the harm-benefit trade-off in prostate cancer screening are more favorable than previous short-term estimates. J Clin Epidemiol 2011;64(12): 1412–7.
12. Pinsky PF, Andriole GL, Kramer BS, et al. Prostate biopsy following a positive screen in the Prostate, Lung, Colorectal and Ovarian cancer screening trial. J Urol 2005;173(3):746–50 [discussion: 50–1].
13. Pinsky PF, Black A, Kramer BS, et al. Assessing contamination and compliance in the prostate

component of the Prostate, Lung, Colorectal, and Ovarian (PLCO) cancer screening trial. Clin Trials 2010;7(4):303–11.

14. Gulati R, Tsodikov A, Wever EM, et al. The impact of PLCO control arm contamination on perceived PSA screening efficacy. Cancer Causes Control 2012; 23(6):827–35.

15. Grubb RL 3rd, Pinsky PF, Greenlee RT, et al. Prostate cancer screening in the Prostate, Lung, Colorectal and Ovarian cancer screening trial: update on findings from the initial four rounds of screening in a randomized trial. BJU Int 2008; 102(11):1524–30.

16. Schröder FH, Denis LJ, Roobol M, et al. The story of the European randomized study of screening for prostate cancer. BJU Int 2003;92(Suppl 2):1–13.

17. Ciatto S, Zappa M, Villers A, et al. Contamination by opportunistic screening in the European randomized study of prostate cancer screening. BJU Int 2003;92(Suppl 2):97–100.

18. Roobol MJ, Kerkhof M, Schröder FH, et al. Prostate cancer mortality reduction by prostate-specific antigen-based screening adjusted for nonattendance and contamination in the European Randomised Study of Screening for Prostate Cancer (ERSPC). Eur Urol 2009;56(4):584–91.

19. Hugosson J, Carlsson S, Aus G, et al. Mortality results from the Goteborg randomised population-based prostate-cancer screening trial. Lancet Oncol 2010;11(8):725–32.

20. Kilpelainen TP, Tammela TL, Malila N, et al. Prostate cancer mortality in the Finnish randomized screening trial. J Natl Cancer Inst 2013;105(10): 719–25.

21. Roobol MJ, Kranse R, Bangma CH, et al. Screening for prostate cancer: results of the Rotterdam Section of the European Randomized Study of Screening for Prostate Cancer. Eur Urol 2013;64(4):530–9.

22. Loeb S, Vonesh EF, Metter EJ, et al. What is the true number needed to screen and treat to save a life with prostate-specific antigen testing? J Clin Oncol 2011;29(4):464–7.

23. Etzioni R, Gulati R, Cooperberg MR, et al. Limitations of basing screening policies on screening trials: the US Preventive Services Task Force and prostate cancer screening. Med Care 2013;51(4):295–300.

24. Heijnsdijk EA, Wever EM, Auvinen A, et al. Quality-of-life effects of prostate-specific antigen screening. N Engl J Med 2012;367(7):595–605.

25. Gulati R, Gore JL, Etzioni R. Comparative effectiveness of alternative prostate-specific antigen-based prostate cancer screening strategies: model estimates of potential benefits and harms. Ann Intern Med 2013;158(3):145–53.

26. Vickers AJ, Ulmert D, Sjoberg DD, et al. Strategy for detection of prostate cancer based on relation between prostate specific antigen at age 40-55 and long term risk of metastasis: case-control study. BMJ 2013;346:f2023.

27. Sox HC. Quality of life and guidelines for PSA screening. N Engl J Med 2012;367(7):669–71.

28. Carter HB, Albertsen PC, Barry MJ, et al. Early detection of prostate cancer: AUA guideline. J Urol 2013;190(2):419–26.

Evolution and Immediate Future of US Screening Guidelines

Kirsten L. Greene, MD, MS*, Sanoj Punnen, MD, MS,
Peter R. Carroll, MD, MPH

KEYWORDS

- Prostate cancer • Screening • Guidelines • Public health • Prostate specific antigen (PSA)

KEY POINTS

- Although observational studies and simulation models have shed some interesting light on many of the uncertainties surrounding prostate cancer screening, well-done clinical trials will provide the best evidence on screening among the extremes of age, the most appropriate interval to screen, and the best complement of tests to use.
- Despite a shift away from expert opinion and favoring more objective methodology such as meta-analysis and systematic review, or perhaps because of it, guidelines can be almost deliberately vague and may be outdated soon after publication.
- Over the last 2 decades, prostate cancer screening has evolved from prioritizing sensitivity of diagnosis in an attempt to favor early detection of localized disease to specificity of detecting men at highest risk with statistically highest benefit.
- Enthusiasm for screening is temporized by acknowledgment that overdetection leads to frequent overtreatment despite evidence supporting the safety of active surveillance in many men with low-risk disease.

HISTORY AND EVOLUTION OF GUIDELINES

The evolution of practice guidelines in medicine has its origin in the early nineteenth century focusing largely on public health measures to control infectious disease epidemics, such as cholera and yellow fever.[1] In the twentieth century, diseases such as tuberculosis and syphilis expanded the role of public health and standardized practices.[2,3] After World War II, the scope of medicine in the United States and Europe expanded rapidly with the development of new drugs and technology. What started as public health mandates moved into the realm of diagnosis and treatment as new therapies for cancer and tuberculosis were developed, including radium and radiographs; these were recognized as potentially dangerous technologies that required protocols for safe use and delivery.[4]

As screening and early detection of different diseases became more ubiquitous, guidelines began to take on the role of cost containment and quality control. Hospitals were targeted as organizations that could be made more efficient by standardizing practice.[5] With so many different treatment options available, both governments and physician groups attempted to unify management as variation came under suspicion for being deviations from standard of care rather than individual judgment heretofore regarded as the "art of medicine."

Department of Urology, UCSF Helen Diller Family Comprehensive Cancer Center, University of California, San Francisco, 1600 Divisadero Street, A631, San Francisco, CA 94115, USA
* Corresponding author. Department of Urology, University of California, San Francisco, 1600 Divisadero Street, Box 1695, San Francisco, CA 94143-1695.
E-mail address: kgreene@urology.ucsf.edu

Urol Clin N Am 41 (2014) 229–235
http://dx.doi.org/10.1016/j.ucl.2014.01.005

Physician groups took on a greater role in guidelines creation in an attempt to maintain physician autonomy.[5]

The American Medical Association played a major role in standardizing medical education, state licensing, and specialty certification in collaboration with specialty societies. The American College of Surgeons began creating uniform standards in surgery by evaluating cancer therapies, standardizing terminology, and publishing results. The American College of Surgeons' first guidelines were published in 1931 addressing fracture care and organizing cancer services in hospitals.[6,7] If guidelines development was slow in the early twentieth century, with 20 guidelines in print by 1945 and 35 more by 1974,[5] publication blossomed in the 1980s and was spurred by organizations advocating cost containment and accountability.[8] In 1989 the Agency for Healthcare Research and Quality was established to produce practice guidelines and currently functions as a guidelines clearinghouse.

In the specialty of Urology, the American Urological Association (AUA) created the Practice Guidelines Committee in 1989 to develop evidence-based guidelines that aim to promote the highest standards of urologic care. The first guideline was introduced in 1994 and addressed the topic of benign prostatic hyperplasia. As evidence-based medicine emerged as a guiding force in education and standardization of medical practice, guidelines development processes changed from expert review of literature and synthesis of recommendations to systematic literature reviews and meta-analysis. Many organizations, including the AUA and European Association of Urology (EAU), have adopted grading systems for the strength of evidence and used this to characterize recommendations.

From 2000 to 2005 the AUA made a set of strategic changes in their guidelines process. This new process optimized cost efficiency of the guidelines process, used the Institute of Medicine criteria, and decreased the creation time of new guidelines from a 5-year process to a 2- to 3-year window. In 2008 the current Level of Recommendation system was implemented to link guidelines statements directly to evidence strength. In 2009, in response to rapidly changing evidence that may render existing guidelines obsolete, the AUA created a new program called the Update Literature Review. Every 15 months a methodologist and 3 panel members, 2 from the original guideline and 1 new member, evaluate new literature to determine if a guideline requires updating.[9] AUA guidelines are published on the Agency for Healthcare Research and Quality's National Guidelines Clearinghouse as well as on the AUA website at auanet.org.

Similarly, the EAU process includes systematic literature review and meta-analysis by a multidisciplinary panel, and grading of evidence based on strength of trial design. Recommendations are based on review of data and panel consensus. Newly published literature is assessed annually to guide future updates.[10]

The National Comprehensive Cancer Center Network guidelines process creates algorithms and decision pathways for management of malignancies based on critical evaluation of current evidence and consensus recommendations by a multidisciplinary panel of experts. Evidence is graded based on the extent, consistency, and quality of data as well as on the level of consensus among the panel and is expressed as categories 1, 2A, 2B, and 3. Uniform consensus requires a majority (85%) of the panel vote. Consensus requires 50% panel vote. The guidelines are continuously reviewed and updated as evidence changes (www.nccn.org).

PROSTATE CANCER SCREENING GUIDELINES

In 1990, the debate over prostate cancer screening surrounded the pros and cons of digital rectal examination (DRE). Half of the cases were detected at a locally advanced stage and still there was debate as to whether there was a survival benefit.[11] Later, the incorporation of prostate-specific antigen (PSA) testing into DRE screening was debated and found to increase overall detection dramatically as well as shift the stage of detection to clinically localized disease.[12]

The AUA released its first Best Practice Statement on prostate cancer screening in 2000. At that time, available data showed that one-third of cancers were diagnosed at a locally advanced or metastatic stage and that "a very large proportion of cancers detected through PSA testing are likely to be clinically important, but that PSA testing is unlikely to detect many of the more prevalent small-volume histologic cancers."[13] Both PSA and DRE were recommended for prostate cancer screening, using a threshold of 4.0 ng/mL, a significant increase in PSA from one test to the next, or an abnormal DRE to prompt consideration of prostate biopsy. The authors recommended a risk-and-benefit discussion with patients and individualization of early detection efforts rather than uniform application of mass screening. Furthermore, testing was recommended to all men age 50 or older with a 10-year life expectancy, and to African American men and those with a family history of prostate cancer in a first-degree relative at an earlier age. This document also addressed the indications for staging tests such as bone scan, PSA kinetics after primary treatment, and PSA behavior in metastatic disease. Methodologically, the Best Practice Policy used literature review, expert opinion, consensus, and peer review.

As the PSA screening era progressed, earlier and more indolent cases were detected and PSA screening came under fire for overdetection and overtreatment of men with prostate cancer. Still, no screening benefit was proven definitively despite attempts at randomized trials to answer this question.[14,15] In 2009 two trials of prostate cancer screening published interim results with different results in terms of the mortality benefit of screening.[16,17] The European Randomized Study of Screening for Prostate Cancer (ERSPC) found a 20% reduction in disease-specific mortality in men screened, whereas the Prostate, Lung, Colorectal, and Ovarian (PLCO) trial found no difference. Both trials came under fire for confounding factors and methodological flaws, which could explain results and both were used by various groups to support their screening recommendations. The results of these trials prompted some groups to encourage prostate cancer screening, including the AUA and American Cancer Society, and others to recommend against it, such as the US Preventive Services Task Force.

The AUA Best Practice Statement was updated in 2009, a year that saw great changes in the level of evidence surrounding PSA screening in the United States and Europe. This publication was similar in methodology to the 2000 document and again used literature review, expert opinion, panel consensus, and peer review. It differed in addressing the interval stage migration of prostate cancer with most cases now being diagnosed at a clinically localized stage. Overdiagnosis and overtreatment of indolent disease were addressed and active surveillance was proposed for patients diagnosed in this category. The age for obtaining a first PSA test was decreased to 40 years in all men with at least a 10-year life expectancy. No threshold PSA was recommended to prompt biopsy and a constellation of factors including free and total PSA, ethnicity, family history, size, age, PSA velocity, and comorbidities were suggested for consideration before proceeding with further testing. Although the guidelines were drafted before the publication of the of the ERSPC and PLCO trials, the authors thought that screening was justified in healthy, well-informed men based on the results of the ERSPC trial.[18]

More recently, the AUA Practice Guidelines Committee changed its methodology to a more formalized evidence-based approach, which uses independently contracted teams of methodologists to perform systematic reviews and meta-analysis of the literature as identified by the expert panel. A strength rating was assigned to the evidence supporting each recommendation ranging from A (high) to C (low). The 2013 Early Detection of Prostate Cancer Guideline differed from the prior 2 documents in both methodology and scope. Recommendations were largely based on modeling studies, meta-analysis, and systematic review of available data more heavily than on expert opinion and consensus, and the document focused on only the use of PSA to screen for prostate cancer rather than including posttreatment PSA kinetics or addressing staging studies.[19]

In summary, the Guideline recommended against screening men younger than age 40 and found no data to support routine screening between 40 and 54 for average-risk men. Similar to the 2009 Best Practice Statements, this Guideline recommended individualization of screening decisions for younger men at higher risk due to race and/or family history. The panel recommended screening for men between 55 and 69 years based on the ERSPC trial but advocated shared decision-making due to the high rate of overdiagnosis and overtreatment. A screening interval of 2 years was suggested rather than annual screening to balance risks and benefits of overdiagnosis and false-positive results. As in the 2000 and 2009 Best Practice Statements, the 2013 Guideline recommends against screening men with less than a 10-year life expectancy but also makes a statement against screening men greater than age 70 due to lack of evidence from modeling and the meta-analysis. A caveat to this is that men in excellent health older than age 70 may benefit from screening.

The primary way to diagnose prostate cancer currently is by transrectal or transperineal prostate biopsy. The risks and benefits of prostate biopsy should be discussed with patients before proceeding. The emergence of fluoroquinolone-resistant *Escherichia coli* has resulted in an increased risk of sepsis from biopsy and is one important possible complication that must be addressed before biopsy.[20,21] The AUA has published a white paper to provide some guidance regarding periprocedural prophylaxis.[22] Along with the infectious risks, hematuria, hematochezia, hematospermia, dysuria and retention, and pain remain concerns that must be carefully considered and weighed against patient comorbidities.[23]

The EAU Early Detection of Prostate Cancer guideline was also updated and released in 2013. The guideline supports PSA screening due to a decrease in prostate cancer–specific mortality, development of advanced disease, and metastasis. This guideline recommends a baseline PSA between ages 40 and 45 years. PSA screening intervals should be based on the baseline PSA level. All men with a life expectancy of at least 10 years should be offered prostate cancer screening.[10]

WHAT ISSUES WILL BE ADDRESSED IN THE IMMEDIATE FUTURE?

The recently issued AUA prostate cancer screening guideline is not without controversy. Others, including the National Comprehensive Cancer Network, will revise guidelines based on new information.

Will Screening Be Supported in the Future?

Although the subject remains controversial, screening is likely to be supported by many. With an extra 2 years of follow-up, from 9 to 11 years, the ERSPC showed that the relative risk reduction of dying from prostate cancer increased from 20% to 38% for screened men versus unscreened men.[16,24] In addition, the number of prostate cancers to detect to save one man from dying of prostate cancer decreased from 48 to 37. As the benefits of screening accrue over time, continued support for screening from level 1 evidence can be expected. The recent AUA guidelines on prostate cancer screening focused on level 1 evidence from randomized trials of screening in making its recommendations.[19] These trials suggested a 20% to 44% relative reduction in prostate cancer death among men ages 55 to 69 years.[16,25]

At What Age Should Screening Start?

There is no level 1 evidence regarding the harms or benefits of screening outside the age range noted above. The AUA suggests that screening in earlier age groups be considered based on risk. However, although screening may be more efficient in high-risk populations, even lower-risk populations could potentially benefit. A recent study by Lilja and colleagues[26] assessed blood from 21,277 Swedish men age 33 to 40. Among the 1312 cases of prostate cancer and 3728 controls without, the authors reported that a single PSA before 50 predicted subsequent prostate cancer up to 30 years later with an AUC of 0.72 (0.75 for advanced prostate cancer). In addition, the risk of prostate cancer death has been shown to be strongly correlated with baseline PSA in men ages 45 to 49 and 51 to 55. In this study, 44% of the deaths in the cohort occurred among men in the highest 10th of the distribution of PSA,

suggesting that there may be a strong rationale for baseline testing in men younger than age 55.[27] The authors contend that early testing can inform an individual about their lifetime risk of prostate cancer and the frequency of which they can be safely screened. However, these men were assessed by only a single PSA before the age of 50, and outcomes of serial screening in such younger populations are unclear, although predictive value has been attributed to a baseline PSA at age 40.[28] Simulation models using national and trial data have suggested that the benefit to screening at an early age is modest.[29] Although rates of overdiagnosis increase only marginally, there is a significant increase in cost and amount of testing. However, if future prospective studies support the observation that screening at an early age may help reduce the number of necessary tests and interval screens, without causing overdiagnosis, and compromising the number of lives saved, a more risk-adapted approach to screening may be seen in the future.

When to Stop Screening?

There is a currently no level 1 evidence to suggest a benefit of screening after age 70.[16,25] A recent study assessing men in the Göteborg trial who were randomized to screening versus no screening until the age of 70 found the benefit of screening faded 9 years after terminating screening.[30] At this point, an equal proportion of lethal cancers were found among screened and unscreened men. Modeling studies have suggested a significant risk of overdetection (50%) with screening older than the age of 70, reflecting that most men older than 70 will have cancer that is unlikely to affect their life expectancy.[31] The Baltimore Longitudinal Study of Aging found that men older than 70 with a PSA lower than 3.0 ng/mL had a low risk of dying of prostate cancer, suggesting they could safely stop screening.[32] Modeling studies looking at another strategy of screening men up to age 74 with an increased threshold for biopsy suggest a reduction in the rate of overdiagnosis by one-third with only a slight impact on lives saved.[29] Only prospective randomized trials assessing the impact of screening in men younger than 55 or older than 70 could determine the true benefit in screening among these age groups. Some point out that the Göteborg trial does address screening in men in the 50 to 55 age range, although only the screening data for men age 55 and older were included in the ERSPC analysis.[25] It is unlikely that such trials will be done, at least in the near future. It should be noted that the results noted above apply to men who have been screened before reaching age 70. Previously unscreened men older than the age of 70 who are in very good health may benefit from at least initial assessment. If screening is undertaken, patients need to be advised, before biopsy, of the significant risk of overdetection.

How Often to Screen?

Although none of the randomized trials were designed to compare various screening intervals, the PLCO randomized men to annual screening versus opportunistic screening, which occurred on average every other year.[17,33] The study found no difference in the risk of death from prostate cancer between groups, suggesting that screening every 2 years may provide comparable survival to screening annually. However, this was not a direct comparison of 2 groups who underwent regular screening at 2 different intervals in a well-conducted randomized trial. Simulation models looking at various screening intervals found that a strategy that screened every other year, with a longer interval (5 years) for men with low PSA levels, found modest differences in lives saved and overdiagnosis, but a large (50%–59%) reduction in the total tests performed and false positives compared with annual screening.[29] Randomized trials comparing men who are randomized to various different screening intervals are required to learn the ideal frequency of screening necessary to maximize survival, while minimizing overdiagnosis and cost from unnecessary testing. However, a 2-year interval seems reasonable.

Should DRE Be Part of Initial Screening?

Although previous studies have suggested a utility for DRE in screening for prostate cancer, its role in more contemporary practice is uncertain. When assessing the control arm of the Prostate Cancer Prevention Trial, a cohort of 5519 men with a normal DRE and PSA less than 3.0 ng/mL, Thompson and colleagues[34] found that an abnormal DRE increased the chance of detecting prostate cancer by almost 2.5-fold.

Recent screening trials have used DRE either in conjunction with PSA for screening[24] or as an ancillary test for patients who are found to have an elevated PSA.[16,25] To elucidate the specific role of DRE in screening for prostate cancer, Gosselaar and colleagues[35] determined the positive predictive value (PPV) of a suspicious and normal DRE within the ERSPC. The authors reported that in conjunction with an elevated PSA ($\geq$30 ng/mL), the PPV at initial screen of a suspicious DRE was 48.6% compared with a PPV of 22.4% for a normal DRE. The PPV decreased for both abnormal and normal DREs on successive screens (screen 2: 29.9% vs 17.1%, screen 3: 21.2% vs 18.2%, respectively). In addition, the authors noted that almost 70% of Gleason 7 cancers detected on each screening interval were found in men with a suspicious DRE, lending support to a beneficial role of DRE in identifying more aggressive tumors.

Because of mixed results from previous studies and the relative paucity of data looking at just DRE alone on screening for prostate cancer, there is still uncertainty regarding the role of DRE as an initial test for prostate cancer screening. DRE may improve the accuracy of detecting more clinically meaningful tumors compared with PSA alone and seems to add little cost or morbidity. However, it can be a barrier to screening for some men and its performance is variable across providers. Therefore, it may be best to consider DRE as optional as a primary screening modality, but it should be done in those found to have an elevated serum PSA.

When to Biopsy?

The AUA guidelines were vague on whom to biopsy, noting that there are many factors to consider. The ERSPC showed a benefit of screening complemented by biopsy of the prostate at a PSA level of 3.0 ng/mL in those 55 years of age or older.[16] If the results of randomized trials are to be followed, this threshold seems reasonable. Others noted, including the AUA, that many factors that may lead to an increased PSA, such as age and prostate volume, be considered instead of relying on an absolute value of PSA alone.[19] Alternatively, risk calculators may be helpful in men who are similar to those in cohorts from which the calculator has been developed.[36,37] Although risk calculators can allow informed decision-making, by reporting the risk of both prostate cancer and aggressive prostate cancer, they are limited by the lack of an evidence-based threshold for when a biopsy should be performed.

Should PSA Velocity Be Used?

The use of PSA velocity to prompt a biopsy is controversial and has not been investigated in randomized clinical trials. Vickers[38] assessed the impact of PSA velocity to predict the likelihood of prostate cancer among 5519 men undergoing biopsy in the control arm of the Prostate Cancer Prevention Trial and found that PSA velocity added very little, in addition to an absolute PSA, to a multivariable model (increase in AUC by 0.07). In addition, it was noted that recommending men solely on PSA velocity without any other indication would lead to a large increase in the number of additional biopsies, with almost 1 in 7 men receiving a biopsy. Further support for this comes from the modeling literature, which found that screening strategies that used PSA velocity were more likely to lead to overdiagnosis and false-positive tests, resulting in more harms relative to incremental lives saved.[31] Although controversy still remains regarding the use of PSA velocity, the concern for false positives and overdetection coupled with a lack of increased predictive accuracy compared with PSA alone has limited its use in contemporary and future guidelines. Randomized trials assessing PSA velocity and other secondary screening tests such as DRE, PSA density, and PCA3 are needed to know the impact of these tests on prostate cancer screening.

SUMMARY

There are many questions left unanswered from the randomized trials on prostate cancer screening. Although observational studies and simulation models have shed some interesting light on many of these uncertainties, well-done clinical trials will provide the best evidence on screening among the extremes of age, the most appropriate interval to screen, and the best complement of tests to use. Despite a shift away from expert opinion and favoring more objective methodology such as meta-analysis and systematic review, or perhaps because of it, guidelines can be almost deliberately vague and may be outdated soon after publication. There is a dearth of high-quality data for analysis so any new study can skew results. Guidelines panels often try to preserve physician autonomy and write guidelines in such a way as to prevent their use in litigation or reimbursement. Over the last 2 decades, prostate cancer screening has evolved from prioritizing sensitivity of diagnosis in an attempt to favor early detection of localized disease to specificity of detecting men at highest risk with statistically highest benefit. Enthusiasm for screening is temporized by acknowledgment that overdetection leads to frequent overtreatment despite evidence supporting the safety of active surveillance in many men with low-risk disease.

REFERENCES

1. Health, B.B.o. Sanitary Measures of the Board of Health (Boston), in Relation to Yellow Fever. 1855.
2. National Tuberculosis Association, Committee on Revision of Diagnostic Standards. Diagnostic standards and classification of tuberculosis. American Trudeau Society; 1955.
3. Buchen JJ. The prevention of venereal disease: with special reference to the report of the British Royal Commission on venereal diseases. Public Health 1917;30:78–86.
4. Dommann M. From danger to risk: the perception and regulation of X-rays in Switzerland. In: Schlich T, Tröhler U, editors. The risks of medical innovation: risk perception and assessment in historical context. London: Routledge; 2006. p. 93–115.
5. Weisz G, Cambrosio A, Keating P, et al. The emergence of clinical practice guidelines. Milbank Q 2007;85(4):691–727.
6. Fracture Committee, American College of Surgeons. The principles and outline of fracture treatment. Bull Am Coll Surg 1931;25(1):3–8.
7. Surgeons, A.C.o., Organization of Service for the Diagnosis and Treatment of Cancer, and minimum standard. 1931.
8. Institute of Medicine. Controlling Costs and Changing Patient Care?. In: The role of utilization management. Washington, DC: National Academy Press; 1989.
9. AUA Resource Manual. A.U. Association. Editor. p. 26–27.
10. Heidenreich A, Bastian PJ, Bellmunt J, et al. EAU guidelines on prostate cancer. Part 1: screening, diagnosis, and local treatment with curative intent—update 2013. Eur Urol 2014;65(1):124–37.
11. Gerber GS, Chodak GW. Digital rectal examination in the early detection of prostate cancer. Urol Clin North Am 1990;17(4):739–44.
12. Cupp MR, Oesterling JE. Prostate-specific antigen, digital rectal examination, and transrectal ultrasonography: their roles in diagnosing early prostate cancer. Mayo Clin Proc 1993;68(3):297–306.
13. Prostate-specific antigen (PSA) best practice policy. American Urological Association (AUA). Oncology (Williston Park) 2000;14(2):267–72, 277–8, 280 passim.
14. Labrie F, Candas B, Dupont A, et al. Screening decreases prostate cancer death: first analysis of the 1988 Quebec prospective randomized controlled trial. Prostate 1999;38(2):83–91.
15. Sandblom G, Varenhorst E, Löfman O, et al. Clinical consequences of screening for prostate cancer: 15 years follow-up of a randomised controlled trial in Sweden. Eur Urol 2004;46(6):717–23 [discussion: 724].
16. Schroder FH, Hugosson J, Roobol MJ, et al. Screening and prostate-cancer mortality in a randomized European study. N Engl J Med 2009; 360(13):1320–8.
17. Andriole GL, Crawford ED, Grubb RL 3rd, et al. Mortality results from a randomized prostate-cancer screening trial. N Engl J Med 2009;360(13):1310–9.

18. Greene KL, Albertsen PC, Babaian RJ, et al. Prostate specific antigen best practice statement: 2009 update. J Urol 2009;182(5):2232–41.

19. Moul JW, Walsh PC, Rendell MS, et al. Early detection of prostate cancer: AUA guideline. J Urol 2013;190(3):1134–7.

20. Laupland KB, Gregson DB, Church DL, et al. Incidence, risk factors and outcomes of Escherichia coli bloodstream infections in a large Canadian region. Clin Microbiol Infect 2008;14(11):1041–7.

21. Carignan A, Roussy JF, Lapointe V, et al. Increasing risk of infectious complications after transrectal ultrasound-guided prostate biopsies: time to reassess antimicrobial prophylaxis? Eur Urol 2012; 62(3):453–9.

22. Wolf JS Jr, Bennett CJ, Dmochowski RR, et al. Best practice policy statement on urologic surgery antimicrobial prophylaxis. J Urol 2008;179(4):1379–90.

23. Berger AP, Gozzi C, Steiner H, et al. Complication rate of transrectal ultrasound guided prostate biopsy: a comparison among 3 protocols with 6, 10 and 15 cores. J Urol 2004;171(4):1478–80 [discussion: 1480–1].

24. Schroder FH, Hugosson J, Roobol MJ, et al. Prostate-cancer mortality at 11 years of follow-up. N Engl J Med 2012;366(11):981–90.

25. Hugosson J, Carlsson S, Aus G, et al. Mortality results from the Goteborg randomised population-based prostate-cancer screening trial. Lancet Oncol 2010;11(8):725–32.

26. Lilja H, Cronin AM, Dahlin A, et al. Prediction of significant prostate cancer diagnosed 20 to 30 years later with a single measure of prostate-specific antigen at or before age 50. Cancer 2011;117(6):1210–9.

27. Vickers AJ, Ulmert D, Sjoberg DD, et al. Strategy for detection of prostate cancer based on relation between prostate specific antigen at age 40–55 and long term risk of metastasis: case-control study. BMJ 2013;346:f2023.

28. Loeb S, Roehl KA, Antenor JA, et al. Baseline prostate-specific antigen compared with median prostate-specific antigen for age group as predictor of prostate cancer risk in men younger than 60 years old. Urology 2006;67(2):316–20.

29. Gulati R, Gore JL, Etzioni R. Comparative effectiveness of alternative prostate-specific antigen–based prostate cancer screening strategies: model estimates of potential benefits and harms. Ann Intern Med 2013;158(3):145–53.

30. Grenabo Bergdahl A, Holmberg E, Moss S, et al. Incidence of prostate cancer after termination of screening in a population-based randomised screening trial. Eur Urol 2013;64(5):703–9.

31. Gulati R, Etzioni R. Alternative prostate cancer screening strategies–in response. Ann Intern Med 2013;158(10):778–9.

32. Schaeffer EM, Carter HB, Kettermann A, et al. Prostate specific antigen testing among the elderly–when to stop? J Urol 2009;181(4):1606–14 [discussion: 1613–4].

33. Hocking WG, Hu P, Oken MM, et al. Lung cancer screening in the randomized Prostate, Lung, Colorectal, and Ovarian (PLCO) Cancer Screening Trial. J Natl Cancer Inst 2010;102(10):722–31.

34. Thompson IM, Ankerst DP, Chi C, et al. Assessing prostate cancer risk: results from the Prostate Cancer Prevention Trial. J Natl Cancer Inst 2006;98(8): 529–34.

35. Pinsky PF, Blacka A, Kramer BS, et al. Assessing contamination and compliance in the prostate component of the Prostate, Lung, Colorectal, and Ovarian (PLCO) Cancer Screening Trial. Clin Trials 2010;7(4):303–11.

36. Ankerst DP, Boeck A, Freedland SJ, et al. Evaluating the Prostate Cancer Prevention Trial High Grade prostate cancer risk calculator in 10 international biopsy cohorts: results from the prostate biopsy collaborative group. World J Urol 2012; 32(1):185–91.

37. van Vugt HA, Kranse R, Steyerberg EW, et al. Prospective validation of a risk calculator which calculates the probability of a positive prostate biopsy in a contemporary clinical cohort. Eur J Cancer 2012; 48(12):1809–15.

38. Vickers AJ. Re: an empirical evaluation of guidelines on prostate-specific antigen velocity in prostate cancer detection. J Natl Cancer Inst 2011;103(21): 1635–6.

International Perspectives on Screening

Monique J. Roobol, PhD, MSc

KEYWORDS

- Prostate cancer • PSA • Screening • Incidence • Mortality • Global

KEY POINTS

- Because cancer, especially prostate cancer (PC), is predominantly a disease of the elderly, increases in the number of older people will inevitably lead to more cases of cancer.
- The worldwide variable relation between prostate cancer mortality and life expectancy points toward racial and dietary influences on the occurrence and characteristics of prostate cancer.
- Contradictory study results are the basis of a still-ongoing debate on whether or not prostate-specific antigen (PSA)–based screening should be offered, which has led to many different guidelines worldwide.
- The PSA test has remarkable features as a screening test (easy to implement, reliable, cheap, capable of risk stratifying men at very low risk), but it is unable to identify men at moderate or high risk of having PC and having a potentially indolent and aggressive PC.
- Worldwide, further research on refining PSA-based algorithms, dealing with overdiagnosis, developing and validating more specific biomarkers, and exploring the role of imaging are ongoing; it is hoped that it will lead to an acceptable prostate cancer screening algorithm.

INTRODUCTION

The estimated population of the world in 2008 was 6.75 billion people, increasing by around 79 million people each year.[1] The world population is aging. In 1970, the world median age was 22 years; and it is projected to reach 38 years by 2050. The number of people in the world aged 60 years and older is expected to almost triple to 2 billion by 2050. Because cancer, especially prostate cancer, is predominantly a disease of the elderly, increases in the number of older people will inevitably lead to more cases of cancer, even if current incidence rates remain the same.[2]

PROSTATE CANCER AND LIFE EXPECTANCY

As early as in 1898, Alberran and Hallé[3] noted the presence of a substantial number of prostate cancers in asymptomatic men. In 1954, Franks[4] described that, in a UK population of men older than 50 years, about 38% harbored a "latent" prostate cancer; already at that time it was mentioned that the observed increase in incidence was caused by lengthening of longevity from 46.6 years in 1911 to 67 years in 1947.

Incidence data of prostate cancer per age group for Europe (United Kingdom) and the United States are shown in **Fig. 1** and confirm these early figures; prostate cancer is a disease of the elderly and, hence, will form a potential health problem for those countries where the life expectancy is relatively high (ie, >70 years).[5]

Similar data are available for prostate cancer mortality (**Fig. 2**). These observations are confirmed when looking at the worldwide distribution of deaths caused by prostate cancer. In 2008, approximately 258,000 men died of prostate cancer, with more than half of these deaths occurring in the developed world.

The relation between life expectancy and age-standardized prostate cancer mortality rates is

Department of Urology, Erasmus University Medical Center, PO Box 2040, Rotterdam 3000 CA, The Netherlands
E-mail address: m.roobol@erasmusmc.nl

Urol Clin N Am 41 (2014) 237–247
http://dx.doi.org/10.1016/j.ucl.2014.01.009

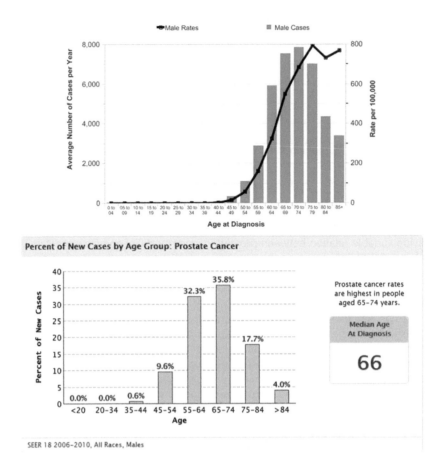

Fig. 1. Prostate cancer incidence per age group (data from the United Kingdom and United States). (*From* Cancer-Stats: cancer statistics for the UK. Available at: http://www.cancerresearchuk.org/cancer-info/cancerstats/ and http://seer.cancer.gov/statfacts/html/prost.html. Accessed January 23, 2014.)

displayed in **Fig. 3**. Remarkable are the Asian and African continent where, in the Asian countries, despite a high life expectancy, the prostate cancer mortality rates are relatively low. It must be noted, however, that the most recent data show an increase.[6] In the African continent, the opposite is true; life expectancy is relatively low, whereas prostate cancer mortality is one of the highest in the world. These observations point toward racial and dietary influences on the occurrence and characteristics of prostate cancer.[6–9] In addition, the availability of structured health care may also play a role.[10]

RANDOMIZED PROSTATE CANCER SCREENING TRIALS

When looking at **Fig. 3**, it is not surprising that studies with the goal to investigate whether population-based screening could reduce prostate cancer–specific mortality were initiated in the United States and Europe.[11,12] Both trials, the European Randomized Study of Screening

for Prostate Cancer (ERSPC) in Europe and the prostate arm of the Prostate, Lung, Colorectal, and Ovarian Cancer Screening Trial (PLCO) in the United States, reported their results on mortality outcomes in 2009 and 2012.[13,14] Remarkably, the results were contradictory. Although the European trial showed a statistically significant relative reduction of 20% in favor of screening, the US trial showed no effect on disease-specific mortality. It is currently generally accepted that the outcome of both trials, being very different in design and conduct, cannot be compared directly. The ERSPC shows an effect of systematic, strictly protocol, prostate-specific antigen (PSA)–based screening versus no screening, whereas the PLCO shows PSA-based screening according to a protocol but with the possibility of including clinical judgment versus a control arm where opportunistic screening was very common.[15,16] Despite these fundamental differences in design both trials, and with the inclusion of smaller (randomized) trials studying the effect of (PSA-based) prostate cancer screening on prostate cancer (PC)

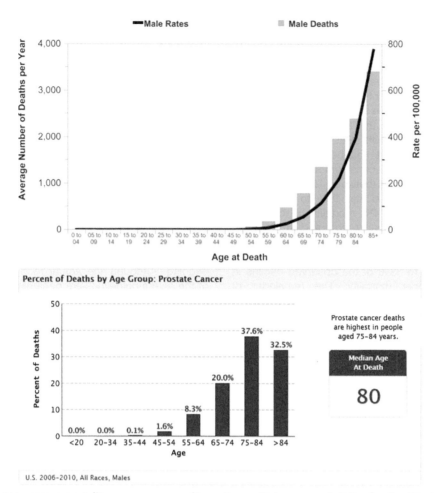

Fig. 2. Prostate cancer mortality per age group. (*From* Cancer-Stats: cancer statistics for the UK. Available at: http://www.cancerresearchuk.org/cancer-info/cancerstats/ and http://seer.cancer.gov/statfacts/html/prost.html. Accessed January 23, 2014.)

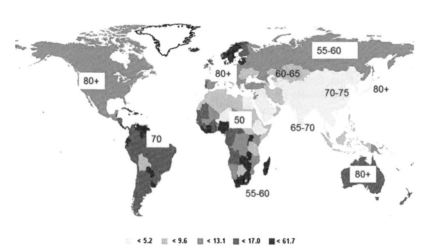

Fig. 3. Life expectancy and estimated age-standardized mortality rate per 100,000 men. (*From* GLOBOCAN 2012: estimated cancer incidence, mortality and prevalence worldwide in 2012. Available at: http://globocan.iarc.fr/. Accessed January 23, 2014.)

mortality, meta-analyses have been performed, which, as can be expected, have been heavily criticized.[17–19]

Next to the randomized prospective trials, modeling studies have been initiated to circumvent the current lack of follow-up and restrictions with respect to sample size. Based on the empiric screening data and the Surveillance, Epidemiology, and End Results (SEER) registry data in the United States, it has been estimated that screening results in a considerable percentage of overdiagnosed cases (between 15% and 37%).[20] The models projected that 45% to 70% of the observed decline in PC mortality in the United States could be plausibly attributed to the stage shift induced by screening. More recent data showed that changes in primary treatment explained 22% to 33% of the observed decline in prostate cancer mortality. The remainder of the decline probably was because of other interventions, such as advances in the treatment of recurrent and progressive disease.[21] When extrapolating the ERSPC mortality reduction to the long-term US setting, it was estimated that the absolute mortality reduction is at least 5 times greater than that observed in the trial with a median follow-up of only 11 years.[22]

Modeling studies can also be used to predict potential harms and benefits of different screening policies.[23] Although the data clearly indicate that PSA screening strategies that use higher thresholds for biopsy referral for older men or screen men with low PSA levels less frequently lead to a reduction in harms, the fact that mortality reduction as compared with more aggressive screening policies is also lowered (although sometimes marginally) further drives uncertainty and debate.[24,25]

GUIDELINES ON PROSTATE CANCER SCREENING

These contradictory and, thus, confusing findings are the basis of a still-ongoing debate on whether or not PSA-based screening should be offered either in the setting of clinical practice (early detection) or in a structured population-based program (screening). This debate has led to many different guidelines worldwide (**Table 1**, adapted/updated from[26]).

Recently, the debate was refueled with the release of updated guidelines on PSA testing by the American Urological Association (AUA).[29] Purely considering the available evidence and addressing both early detection and screening asymptomatic men, the panel recommends against PSA testing in men younger than 40 years.

The panel does not recommend routine screening in men aged between 40 and 54 years at average risk; for men aged 55 to 69 years, the panel recommends shared decision making. In addition, the panel advises a 2-year or more screening interval to reduce the harms of screening and intervals for rescreening to be individualized by a baseline PSA level in men with more than average risk on developing PC. With respect to the upper age cutoff for screening, no routine PSA screening in men aged 70 years and older or any man with less than a 10- to 15-year life expectancy is advised. However, men aged 70 years and older who are in excellent health may benefit from prostate cancer screening. As expected, similar to the ongoing debate on the 2 randomized trials, these guidelines resulted in a fierce debate, which is still ongoing. Although the actual recommendations of the AUA's guidelines are generally accepted, it is more the way they are presented and, hence, interpreted.[35] The 5 statements primarily address asymptomatic men and as a result recommendations applying to men at higher risk appear to have been lost in the emphasis. Altogether these contradictory scientific publications, editorials, guidelines, and public discussions are extremely confusing for both clinicians and laypeople. The worldwide urological association (Societe International d'Urologie) has, to be of aid in this dilemma, released 3 decision aids for urologists, general practitioners (GPs), and laypeople.[36] It is obvious that an important task awaits the scientists working on prostate cancer screening and early detection and that this controversy, leading to uncertainty, needs to be resolved as soon as possible.

SCREENING INITIATIVES WORLDWIDE

Meanwhile, around the world national screening studies/programs are being initiated. Studies initiated with the goal to study more advanced state-of-the-art screening algorithms or with the goal to assess feasibility and performance characteristics in their specific national settings.

Population-Based Screening in Lithuania, the Early Prostate Cancer Detection Program

Despite the uncertainties mentioned earlier, the Lithuanian Ministry of Health, already in 2006, launched the national Early Prostate Cancer Detection Program (EPCDP).[37] According to the regulations of the EPCDP, men aged 50 to 75 years attending GPs are informed about the possibilities of early detection of PC and offered a PSA test free of charge once a year. This service is also offered to men aged 45 to 49 years if their first-degree

Table 1
Guidelines and recommendations on prostate cancer screening

Guideline Group	Recommendation	Age to Begin	Interval/Algorithm
US Preventive Services Task Force	Recommends against screening (grade D)	—	—
American Cancer Society	Informed decision making	Begin PSA testing at 40 y if at highest risk (several first-degree relatives diagnosed with prostate cancer <65 y). Begin at 45 y for men at high risk (African American men and/or men with a first-degree relative). "Begin at age 50 for men at average risk and with a life-expectancy >10 y."	"Men who choose to be tested who have a PSA of less than 2.5 ng/mL, may only need to be retested every 2 y." "Screening should be done yearly for men whose PSA level is 2.5 ng/mL or higher."
American Urological Association	Well-informed men who wish to pursue early diagnosis	There should be no PSA screening in men younger than 40 y. There should be no routine screening in men aged between 40 and 54 y at average risk. There should be shared decision making for men aged 55 to 69 y who are considering PSA screening, and proceed based on a man's values and preferences. There should be no routine PSA screening in men aged 70+ y or any man with less than a 10- to 15-y life expectancy.	There should be a routine screening interval of 2 y or more, individualized by a baseline PSA level.
European Association of Urology	Insufficient evidence to recommend widespread population-based PSA screening Early detection (opportunistic screening) offered to well-informed men	There should be a baseline PSA at 40 y.	Base the subsequent screening interval on the baseline PSA. A screening interval of 8 y might be enough in men with initial PSA levels <1 ng/mL. Further PSA testing is not necessary in men older than 75 y and a baseline PSA <3 ng/mL because of their very low risk of dying of prostate cancer.
National Comprehensive Cancer Network	Informed discussion	There should be baseline DRE and PSA at 40 y. There should be annual screening at 50 y.	The algorithm is based on initial testing. Repeat screening at 45 y of age if the PSA is <1.0 ng/mL.

(continued on next page)

Table 1
(continued)

Guideline Group	Recommendation	Age to Begin	Interval/Algorithm
American College of Preventive Medicine	Insufficient evidence to recommend routine screening	Discussion about screening should occur annually, during the routine periodic examination, or in response to a request by patients.	—
Melbourne Consensus Statement	Routine population-based screening not recommended	Healthy, well-informed men (aged 55–69 y) should be fully counseled about the positive and negative aspects of PSA testing to reduce their risk of metastases and death; a baseline PSA in the 40s has value for risk stratification. All should be part of the shared decision-making process.	—
Japanese Urological Association	Recommends PSA screening	Candidates for PSA screening are men aged 50 y or older in general and 40 y or older in men with a family history.	The optimal screening interval cannot be stated at present but might be closely related to baseline PSA levels; it should be once every 3 y for men with baseline PSA levels lower than 1.0 ng/mL and annually for men with baseline PSA levels >1.0 ng/mL.

Abbreviation: DRE, digital rectal examination.
  Data from Refs.[27–34]

relatives have PC. Health care providers are not prompted or supported to invite men for PSA testing, though this approach is not forbidden. Men participating in EPCPD are informed by GPs about the benefits and pitfalls of PSA testing. Participants must sign an informed consent form before inclusion into the program. GPs refer participants for further workup if the PSA is greater than 3 ng/mL. The decision to perform prostate biopsy is at the discretion of the patient and consulting urologist. The main objectives of the EPCDP are to increase detection of PC at an early stage and to reduce mortality of patients with PC. So far, Lithuania is the only country in Europe to offer PSA testing to healthy asymptomatic men. A recent publication shows that after the introduction of the EPCDP in Lithuania, the incidence of PC reached 227.8 per 100,000 in 2006 to 2008 and is now among the highest in Europe. An effect on PC mortality has not yet been observed with limited follow-up. The program is ongoing.[38]

The Stockholm 2–3 Project

Stockholm (STHLM) 2 is the largest research project in Sweden about prostate cancer and is a collaboration between Karolinska Institutet and Karolinska University Hospital. The aim is to find how heredity, environment, and genetic changes can be used to predict the risk of developing prostate cancer. A total of 26,000 men who were visiting a physician and took a PSA test or were diagnosed with PC in the Stockholm health care system were included in this bio bank initiative (2010–2012). Men contributed samples of DNA, plasma, and urine and were also asked to fill out a Web questionnaire about lifestyle factors. The collected material and data will be analyzed with respect to their capability to predict PC yes or no, and even more important to ability to predict potentially aggressive PC. Analyses will be based on promising serum biomarker panels and/or available genomic markers in combination with detailed follow-up on incidence and mortality. The next step is the new project STHLM3 starting in 2013. The aim of STHLM3 is a systemized prostate cancer testing for all men within the age range of 50 to 69 years in the Stockholm area. Approximately 260,000 men will be invited and randomized to either a control/PSA arm whereby referral to biopsy will be based on PSA only, with a PSA of 3 or greater as the level of referral to prostate biopsy, and an intervention/best biomarker panel arm whereby referral to biopsy will be determined by a risk prediction model based on age, an array of single-nucleotide polymorphisms (SNPs), family history, and protein-based biomarkers.[39]

The Prostate Cancer Risk Management Program in the United Kingdom

In the United Kingdom, there is no organized screening program for PC, but there is an informed choice program. The aim of the Prostate Cancer Risk Management program is to ensure that men who are concerned about the risk of prostate cancer receive clear and balanced information about the advantages and disadvantages of the PSA test and treatment of prostate cancer. This information will help men to decide whether they want to have the test. Their statement is that any man older than 50 years who asks for a PSA test after careful consideration of the implications should be given one.[40]

Within the so-called ProtecT trial (evaluating the effectiveness of treatment for clinically localised prostate cancer) in the UK there is a sub-study called The CAP (Comparison Arm for ProtecT) study. The objective of this study is to evaluate the effectiveness of population screening for PC by establishing a cluster randomised trial allocating general practices to either intensive case-finding (the ProtecT trial) or unscreened standard practice in order to: provide an unbiased estimate of the effect of a single screening round for PC on PC-specific and all-cause mortality in the population, and to contribute to the international effort to investigate the impact of PC screening.[41] Both studies are ongoing and are expected to report their findings in 2015.[41]

PSA-Based Screening or Risk-Based Screening, Individual Risk Assessment for Prostate Cancer: an Impact Analysis, the Netherlands

PSA-based early detection/screening is far from perfect. The performance characteristics of the PSA test leads to unnecessary testing, the diagnosis of potentially indolent PC, and subsequent overtreatment. This circumstance has led to numerous approaches to improve predictive

capability. One of these approaches is to combine the outcome of the PSA test with other relevant prebiopsy information into so-called risk calculators or nomograms. These multivariate risk stratification tools hold great potential for screening prostate cancer as well as for diagnosing, classifying, and monitoring this disease.[42–44] Although their potential to be of aid in reducing unnecessary testing and overdiagnosis is, thus, well known, accepted actual use of these prediction tools in clinical practice is not common. A recent survey among oncologists and urologists reported that 55% of the urologists actually used prostate cancer nomograms.[45] In the Netherlands, an implementation study was initiated with the goal to stimulate the use of the Rotterdam prostate cancer risk calculator[46,47] into clinical practice. A total of 5 Dutch urological clinics participated, and 443 men were included in this study whereby a prostate biopsy was recommended if the calculated risk was 20% or more.[48] Both urologists and patients complied with the risk calculator (RC) recommendation in 83% of the cases. If a biopsy was recommended, almost all patients (96%) complied, although 36% of patients with a calculated risk less than 20% were biopsied. Noteworthy was the fact that if urologists opted for biopsies against the recommendations of the RC (calculated risk <20%), it was because of an elevated PSA level ($\geq$3 ng/mL). In addition, the RC predicted outcome of prostate biopsy better than basing the decision to biopsy on the outcome of PSA and the outcome of the digital rectal examination (DRE); the positive predictive value (PPV, ie, the number of prostate biopsies with PC detected divided by the total number of prostate biopsies) using a risk cutoff of 20% or more was 49%.[49] This active implementation study (providing support of a study nurse during the clinic) has shown that the use of a risk-based approach is well accepted by both urologists and patients and that the number of unnecessary biopsies can be reduced. The challenge now is to continue and expand the use of these tools in clinical practice.

PSA Mass Screening in the Federal State of Tyrol, Austria

The objective of this trial initiated in 1993 was to monitor the impact of screening in a natural experiment by comparing prostate cancer mortality in Tyrol, where PSA testing was introduced at no charge, with the rest of Austria, where it was not introduced.

This mass screening project was conducted between October 1993 and September 1994 with

PSA as the initial test for the early detection of prostate carcinoma. Approximately 65,000 Tyrolean males age 45–75 years were invited to participate in this screening program free of charge. Twenty-one thousand and seventy-eight male volunteers (32%) responded. Of the 21,078 volunteers, 1618 (8%) had elevated PSA levels according to age-referenced levels. Of these men, 778 (48%) underwent biopsies; 197 biopsies (25%) were positive for PC.

In the latest publication[50] of the Tyrol trial applying an age-period-cohort model using Poisson regression, to the mortality data covering more than three decades from 1970 to 2008 it was found that there was a significant reduction in PC mortality with a risk ratio of 0.70 (95% confidence interval 0.57, 0.87) for Tyrol, and for Austria excluding Tyrol a moderate reduction with a risk ratio of 0.92 (95% confidence interval 0.87, 0.97), each compared to the mortality rate in the period 1989–1993.

The conclusions from the study were that the decline in prostate cancer mortality was probably due to aggressive down staging and successful treatment.

PSA-Based Screening in Asia

In a recent report from a multidisciplinary panel from Asia-Pacific countries that met during a consensus session on prostate cancer (2013 Asian Oncology Summit in Bangkok, Thailand), it became clear that there is a general trend toward an increasing incidence of prostate cancer in countries, such as China, Japan, the Philippines, Singapore, South Korea, and Thailand.[51] However, because of the lack of high-level evidence on the effectiveness of PSA-based screening pertaining to the Asian population, the committee stresses the need for local studies to validate the European and US guidelines.

One of the largest initiatives was a PSA-based screening trial in China. From July 1999 to April 2002, a total of 19,808 Chinese men in Changchun who were older than 50 years were invited for screening.[52] A total of 12,027 men agreed to participate.[51] The PSA distribution and, hence, the cancer detection rate (CDR) was quite different from the European and US data. Ninety-three percent of men had a PSA less than 4.0 ng/mL. A total of 158 men were actually biopsied, resulting in 41 PC cases detected (PPV 25.9% and CDR 0.34%). Gleason grading of the PC found that 22% of PC were Gleason 6. The investigators concluded that although PSA distribution differs from the Western world, the PPV and the relationship of PSA, CDR, and Gleason grading is comparable.

This last observation is confirmed by a Japanese study whereby PPVs per PSA level were assessed.[53] The study cohort consisted of men with initial PSA levels less than 4.0 ng/mL and no suspicious findings on DRE from a population-based prostate cancer screening cohort in Gunma Prefecture, Japan and ERSPC section Rotterdam. Looking at a 4-year period, the investigators concluded that the risk of developing PC was greater for Dutch men because they had higher initial PSA levels. However, there was no significant difference in PC risk between Dutch and Japanese men whose baseline PSA levels fall within the same range.

The Japanese cohort used in the study mentioned earlier originated from the Gunma PSA-based screening study.[54] The Gunma study was initiated in 1981. Between 1981 and 1991, DRE and prostatic acid phosphatase were used as screening modalities. After 1992, PSA-based screening has been carried out for all participants. DRE and transrectal ultrasonography were also performed as ancillary tests in most municipalities until 1994. Between 1992 and 2000, 13,021 men, 50 to 79 years old, had their PSA level measured. Similar to the Chinese data, 92.6% had an initial PSA level of 4.0 ng/mL or less. In this particular study of the Gunma cohort, the focus was on PSA change and confirmed earlier observations that the probability of PSA increase toward PSA levels greater than 4.0 ng/mL was similar between Americans and Japanese men having the same baseline PSA ranges.

More recent data from Japan come from a PSA-based screening system for PC initiated by the municipal government in Kanazawa.[55] In the 2000–2005 period, a total of 27,730 men aged 55 to 69 years were PSA tested. From 2000 to 2002, patients with total PSA (tPSA) greater than 2.1 ng/mL were referred for further assessment. Since 2003, patients with tPSA levels ranging from 2.1 to 10.0 ng/mL and free/tPSA ratios more than 0.22 have not been referred. Although 2810 men were further assessed, only 925 men were actually biopsied (based on clinical judgment and DRE) and 214 PC were detected. During the 6-year period, 60 of the 214 men with PC had PSA levels between 2.1 and 4.0 ng/mL.

With this last observation, the investigators confirm the US and European data showing that, at low PSA values, PC is also present at considerable rates.[56,57]

SUMMARY

PC screening has been one of the most controversial topics in the urological society for decades.

Although the PSA test has remarkable features as a screening test (easy to implement, reliable, cheap, capable of risk stratifying men at very low risk), it is hampered by a lack of identifying men at moderate or high risk of having PC; in addition, it cannot distinguish between potentially indolent and aggressive PC. In PC screening, the latter is especially of crucial importance; PC is a disease with different faces and is very common, especially in older men. This point automatically implies that screening for PC with the PSA test will coincide with unnecessary testing and the diagnosis of PC cases that, without being detected, would never cause any complaints before death. This unnecessary testing and overdiagnosis are the basis of the ongoing debate on whether screening or early detection for PC is indicated and should be pursued at a large scale. Currently, there is no solution for this dilemma. Worldwide, there is ample research ongoing showing that, in general, PC incidence is increasing. However, worldwide studies all show similarity with respect to the performance characteristics of the PSA test. Worldwide, further research on refining PSA-based algorithms, dealing with overdiagnosis, developing and validating more specific biomarkers, and exploring the role of imaging are ongoing; it is hoped that it will lead to an answer to this frequently asked question: Should we screen for PC? For now, we are obliged to inform our peers and potential patients as well as possible to be sure that if one applies or undergoes PSA screening, it is with full knowledge of all potential harms and benefits.

REFERENCES

1. UN. World population prospects: the 2008 revision. New York: United Nations, Department of Economic and Social Affairs, Population Division; 2009.
2. Available at: http://publications.cancerresearchuk.org. Accessed June 1, 2013.
3. Alberran J, Hallé N. Hypertrophie et néoplasies épitheliales de la prostate. Ann des Mal. Org. Gen-Urin 1898;17:797–801.
4. Franks LM. Latent carcinoma of the prostate. J Pathol Bacteriol 1954;68:603–16.
5. Available at: http://seer.cancer.gov/statfacts/html/prost.html. Accessed February 13, 2014.
6. Namiki M, Akaza H, Lee SE, et al. Prostate cancer working group report. Jpn J Clin Oncol 2010; 40(Suppl 1):i70–5.
7. Akaza H, Hinotsu S, Cooperberg MR, et al. Sixth joint meeting of J-CaP and CaPSURE–a multinational perspective on prostate cancer management and patient outcomes. Jpn J Clin Oncol 2013; 43(7):756–66.
8. Kinseth MA, Jia Z, Rahmatpanah F, et al. Expression between African American and Caucasian prostate cancer tissue reveals that stroma is the site of aggressive changes. Int J Cancer 2014; 134(1):81–91.
9. Chu LW, Ritchey J, Devesa SS, et al. Prostate cancer incidence rates in Africa. Prostate Cancer 2011;2011:947870.
10. Stokes WA, Hendrix LH, Royce TJ, et al. Racial differences in time from prostate cancer diagnosis to treatment initiation: a population-based study. Cancer 2013;119(13):2486–93.
11. Schröder FH, Hugosson J, Roobol MJ, et al, ERSPC Investigators. Screening and prostate-cancer mortality in a randomized European study. N Engl J Med 2009;360(13):1320–8.
12. Andriole GL, Crawford ED, Grubb RL 3rd, et al, PLCO Project Team. Mortality results from a randomized prostate-cancer screening trial. N Engl J Med 2009;360(13):1310–9.
13. Andriole GL, Crawford ED, Grubb RL 3rd, et al, PLCO Project Team. Prostate cancer screening in the randomized prostate, lung, colorectal, and ovarian cancer screening trial: mortality results after 13 years of follow-up. J Natl Cancer Inst 2012; 104(2):125–32.
14. Schröder FH, Hugosson J, Roobol MJ, et al, ERSPC Investigators. Prostate-cancer mortality at 11 years of follow-up. N Engl J Med 2012; 366(11):981–90.
15. Schröder FH, Roobol MJ. ERSPC and PLCO prostate cancer screening studies: what are the differences? Eur Urol 2010;58(1):46–52.
16. Gulati R, Tsodikov A, Wever EM, et al. The impact of PLCO control arm contamination on perceived PSA screening efficacy. Cancer Causes Control 2012;23(6):827–35.
17. Ilic D, Neuberger MM, Djulbegovic M, et al. Screening for prostate cancer. Cochrane Database Syst Rev 2013;(1):CD004720.
18. Djulbegovic M, Beyth RJ, Neuberger MM, et al. Screening for prostate cancer: systematic review and meta-analysis of randomised controlled trials. BMJ 2010;341:c4543.
19. Roobol MJ, Carlsson S, Hugosson J. Meta-analysis finds screening for prostate cancer with PSA does not reduce prostate cancer-related or all-cause mortality but results likely due to heterogeneity - the two highest quality studies identified do find prostate cancer-related mortality reductions. Evid Based Med 2011;16(1):20–1.
20. Etzioni R, Tsodikov A, Mariotto A, et al. Quantifying the role of PSA screening in the US prostate cancer mortality decline. Cancer Causes Control 2008; 19(2):175–81.
21. Etzioni R, Gulati R, Tsodikov A, et al. The prostate cancer conundrum revisited: treatment changes

and prostate cancer mortality declines. Cancer 2012;118(23):5955–63.

22. Etzioni R, Gulati R, Cooperberg MR, et al. Limitations of basing screening policies on screening trials: the US preventive services task force and prostate cancer screening. Med Care 2013;51(4): 295–300.

23. Gulati R, Gore JL, Etzioni R. Comparative effectiveness of alternative prostate-specific antigen–based prostate cancer screening strategies: model estimates of potential benefits and harms. Ann Intern Med 2013; 158(3):145–53.

24. Summaries for patients. Screening smarter, not harder, for prostate cancer. Ann Intern Med 2013; 158(3):1–30.

25. Concato J. Probability, uncertainty, and prostate cancer. Ann Intern Med 2013;158(3):211–2.

26. Roobol MJ, Carlsson SV. Risk stratification in prostate cancer screening. Nat Rev Urol 2013;10(1): 38–48.

27. Moyer VA, U.S. Preventive Services Task Force. Screening for prostate cancer: U.S. preventive services task force recommendation statement. Ann Intern Med 2012;157(2):120–34.

28. Wolf AM, Wender RC, Etzioni RB, et al. American Cancer Society guideline for the early detection of prostate cancer: update 2010. CA Cancer J Clin 2010;60:70–98.

29. Carter HB, Albertsen PC, Barry MJ, et al. Early detection of prostate cancer: AUA guideline. J Urol 2013;190(2):419–26.

30. Heidenreich A, Bellmunt J, Bolla M, et al. EAU guidelines on prostate cancer. Part 1: screening, diagnosis, and treatment of clinically localised disease. Eur Urol 2011;59:61–71.

31. Kawachi MH, Bahnson RR, Barry M, et al. NCCN clinical practice guidelines in oncology: prostate cancer early detection. J Natl Compr Canc Netw 2010;8:240–62.

32. Lim LS, Sherin K. Screening for prostate cancer in U.S. men ACPM position statement on preventive practice. Am J Prev Med 2008;34:164–70.

33. Murphy DG, Ahlering T, Catalona WJ, et al. The Melbourne consensus statement on the early detection of prostate cancer. BJU Int 2014;113(2): 186–8.

34. The Committee for Establishment of the Guidelines on Screening for Prostate Cancer, Japanese Urological Association. Updated Japanese Urological Association Guidelines on prostate-specific antigen-based screening for prostate cancer in 2010. Int J Urol 2010;17(10):830–8.

35. Available at: http://www.bjuinternational.com/bjui-blog/the-new-aua-psa-testing-guidelines-leave-me-scratching-my-head/. Accessed January 10, 2014.

36. Available at: http://www.siu-urology.org/psa-aid. aspx. Accessed January 10, 2014.

37. Jankevicius F, Adomaitis R, Jievaltas M, et al. The launch of the Lithuanian Early Prostate Cancer Detection Program (EPCDP). Eur Urol Suppl 2007;6:174.

38. Smailyte G, Aleknaviciene B. Incidence of prostate cancer in Lithuania after introduction of the Early Prostate Cancer Detection Programme. Public Health 2012;126:1075–7.

39. Available at: http://controlled-trials.com/ISRCTN 84445406. Accessed June 16, 2013.

40. Available at: http://www.cancerscreening.nhs.uk/ prostate/index.html. Accessed June 16, 2013.

41. Lane JA, Hamdy FC, Martin RM, et al. Latest results from the UK trials evaluating prostate cancer screening and treatment: the CAP and ProtecT studies. Eur J Cancer 2010;46(17): 3095–101.

42. Iremashvili V, Soloway MS, Pelaez L, et al. Comparative validation of nomograms predicting clinically insignificant prostate cancer. Urology 2013;81(6): 1202–8.

43. Nguyen CT, Kattan MW. Formalized prediction of clinically significant prostate cancer: is it possible? Asian J Androl 2012;14(3):349–54.

44. Zhu X, Albertsen PC, Andriole GL, et al. Risk-based prostate cancer screening [review]. Eur Urol 2012;61(4):652–61.

45. Kim SP, Karnes RJ, Nguyen PL, et al. Clinical implementation of quality of life instruments and prediction tools for localized prostate cancer: results from a national survey of radiation oncologists and urologists. J Urol 2013;189(6):2092–8.

46. Kranse R, Roobol M, Schroder FH. A graphical device to represent the outcomes of a logistic regression analysis. Prostate 2008;68:1674–80.

47. Roobol MJ, Steyerberg EW, Kranse R, et al. A risk-based strategy improves prostate-specific antigen-driven detection of prostate cancer. Eur Urol 2010; 57:79–85.

48. van Vugt HA, Roobol MJ, Busstra M, et al. Compliance with biopsy recommendations of a prostate cancer risk calculator. BJU Int 2012;109(10): 1480–8.

49. van Vugt HA, Kranse R, Steyerberg EW, et al. Prospective validation of a risk calculator which calculates the probability of a positive prostate biopsy in a contemporary clinical cohort. Eur J Cancer 2012; 48(12):1809–15.

50. Oberaigner W, Siebert U, Horninger W, et al. Prostate-specific antigen testing in Tyrol, Austria: prostate cancer mortality reduction was supported by an update with mortality data up to 2008. Int J Public Health 2012;57(1):57–62.

51. Williams S, Chiong E, Lojanapiwat B, et al. Management of prostate cancer in Asia: resource-stratified guidelines from the Asian Oncology Summit 2013. Lancet Oncol 2013;14:e524–34.

52. Gao HE, Li YL, Wu S, et al. Mass screening of prostate cancer in a Chinese population: the relationship between pathological features of prostate cancer and serum prostate specific antigen. Asian J Androl 2005;7(2):159–63.

53. Ito K, Raaijmakers R, Roobol M, et al. Prostate carcinoma detection and increased prostate-specific antigen levels after 4 years in Dutch and Japanese males who had no evidence of disease at initial screening. Cancer 2005;103(2): 242–50.

54. Ito K, Yamamoto T, Ohi M, et al. Cumulative probability of PSA increase above 4.0 ng/ml in population based screening for prostate cancer. Int J Cancer 2004;109:455–60.

55. Kobori Y, Kitagawa Y, Mizokami A, et al. Free-to-total prostate-specific antigen (PSA) ratio contributes to an increased rate of prostate cancer detection in a Japanese population screened using a PSA level of 2.1–10.0 ng/ml as a criterion. Int J Clin Oncol 2008; 13:229–32.

56. Bul M, van Leeuwen PJ, Zhu X, et al. Prostate cancer incidence and disease-specific survival of men with initial prostate-specific antigen less than 3.0 ng/ml who are participating in ERSPC Rotterdam. Eur Urol 2011;59:498–505.

57. Thompson IM, Pauler DK, Goodman PJ, et al. Prevalence of prostate cancer among men with a prostate specific antigen level ≤4.0 ng per ml. N Engl J Med 2004;350:2239–46.

The Politics of Prostate Cancer Screening

Samuel D. Kaffenberger, MD[a],
David F. Penson, MD, MPH[b,c],*

KEYWORDS

- Prostate cancer • Localized • Screening • Prostate-specific antigen
- United States Preventive Services Task Force

KEY POINTS

- There is a perception among policymakers that effective screening programs that identify patients at high risk for a disease or diagnose a condition earlier in its disease course may result in reduced health care costs.
- Much disagreement exists among government agencies, payers, and policymakers concerning whether prostate cancer screening using the prostate-specific antigen test should be a component of routine preventive health care maintenance for American men.
- In the case of the United States Preventive Services Task Force (USPSTF), one can argue that politics plays a role in the development of guidelines, and that this has influenced their recommendation concerning prostate cancer screening.
- Efforts are currently under way to improve the efficiency and transparency of the USPSTF in the form of the USPSTF Transparency and Accountability Act of 2013.
- It is of particular importance that urologists have a voice in the creation of health policy for conditions that we directly diagnose and treat.

Preventive screenings are recognized as an important part of routine health care maintenance and are routinely promoted by governmental agencies, such as the Centers for Disease Control and Prevention, the Agency for Healthcare Research and Quality (AHRQ), and the National Institutes of Health. There is a general perception among policymakers that effective screening programs that identify patients at high risk for a disease or diagnose a condition earlier in its disease course may result in reduced health care costs down the line. In the case of cancer, while primary prevention through behavior modification or other interventions is most desirable, it is often not feasible and, as such, the goal of most cancer screening interventions tends to be secondary prevention, identifying the malignancy earlier in the disease course and rapidly initiating effective therapies that affect outcomes. The last clause of this sentence is critical, as a screening program that identifies a disease at an earlier stage but does not ultimately reduce morbidity and/or mortality would be considered ineffective and a waste of limited health care resources. An example of an effective cancer screening intervention that has been widely endorsed by payers, government agencies, and policymakers is the regular use of the Papanicolaou (Pap) test to screen for cervical cancer. Because there is solid evidence that the Pap test identifies cervical cancer at an earlier stage and

Source of funding: None.
[a] Department of Urologic Surgery, Vanderbilt University, 2525 West End Avenue, Nashville, TN, USA; [b] Department of Urologic Surgery, VA Tennessee Valley Geriatric Research, Education, and Clinical Center (GRECC), Vanderbilt University, 2525 West End Avenue, Nashville, TN, USA; [c] Center for Surgical Quality and Outcomes Research, Vanderbilt University, 2525 West End Avenue, Suite 1200, Nashville, TN 37203-1738, USA
* Corresponding author. Center for Surgical Quality and Outcomes Research, Vanderbilt University, 2525 West End Avenue, Suite 1200, Nashville, TN 37203-1738.
E-mail address: david.penson@vanderbilt.edu

Urol Clin N Am 41 (2014) 249–255
http://dx.doi.org/10.1016/j.ucl.2014.01.004
0094-0143/14/$ – see front matter Published by Elsevier Inc.

also that morbidity and mortality from the disease are reduced as a result of testing,[1] there is no controversy surrounding the use of or payment for this test in cervical cancer screening.

Inherent in any discussion concerning screening policies is a natural tension that develops between making population-wide recommendations concerning a health care intervention and advising individual patients in the setting of clinical decision making. As urologists, we are trained to view and treat each patient individually, and to consider unique preferences concerning outcomes when counseling patients regarding clinical decisions. By contrast, however, policymakers consider health care interventions at the level of the population, balancing the harms and benefits of a screening program in the aggregate. This approach can result in a population-level recommendation that may be in conflict with an individual patient's preferences and desires. This conflict holds particularly true in a situation where a screening intervention is shown to have a positive effect on disease-related morbidity and/or mortality, but is also associated with a set of harms that may outweigh the benefits of early detection. Such is the case in prostate cancer screening, where there is evidence that screening clearly allows us to detect the disease at an earlier stage and reduces mortality,[2] but where there exists great controversy regarding whether the morbidity and mortality benefits of screening outweigh the harms. In turn this has resulted in disagreement between government agencies, payers, and policymakers concerning whether prostate cancer screening, using the prostate-specific antigen (PSA) test, should be a component of routine preventive health care maintenance for American men.

The various organizations that generate guidelines regarding PSA screening have major differences in perspective (population vs individual) that are reflected in their approach to developing these guidelines. For example, organizations such as the National Comprehensive Cancer Network and the European Association of Urology use a consensus process for setting guidelines,[3,4] based primarily on expert opinion and interpretation of the available literature. This approach is consistent with the fact that these organizations consist primarily of providers and the goal of their guidelines is to provide insight into the treatment of individual patients. By contrast, organizations such as the United States Preventive Services Taskforce (USPSTF), the American Urological Association, and the American Cancer Society use a different, evidence-based approach to the development of guidelines.[5,6] In the particular

case of the USPSTF, however, one can argue that politics plays a role in the development of guidelines and that this influenced their recommendation concerning prostate cancer screening. This article discusses the history of the USPSTF and how it arrived at its recommendation, and suggests future advocacy efforts that will result in a more inclusive guidelines process.

THE HISTORY AND MISSION OF THE USPSTF

Originally formed in 1984, the USPSTF is a government-appointed panel of 16 volunteer members, each serving a 4-year term.[5] Members of the panel are appointed by the director of the AHRQ (1 of 12 agencies under the auspices of the US Department of Health and Human Services) with the guidance of the Chair and Vice-Chair of the Task Force. Although the task force is funded by AHRQ, it operates quasi-independently of this agency, in that it receives funding and administrative support from AHRQ, but the agency has no further oversight in the decision-making process. The task force members are gathered from the fields of primary care and preventive medicine, including family medicine, internal medicine, pediatrics, obstetrics and gynecology, behavioral health, and nursing. Noteworthy is that no specialty fields are represented on the panel.

The stated mission of the USPSTF is "to evaluate the benefits of individual services based on age, gender, and risk factors for disease; make recommendations about which preventive services should be incorporated routinely into primary medical care and for which populations; and identify a research agenda for clinical preventive care."[5] It is worth noting that the USPSTF is specifically prohibited from assessing the cost-effectiveness of the preventive services it evaluates. The services or topics that are evaluated are chosen by the USPSTF from public nominations (available at http://www.uspreventive servicestaskforce.org/tftopicnon.htm) at 1 of 3 annual USPSTF meetings. The public can nominate a new topic for consideration or suggest reconsideration of a previously evaluated topic because of availability of new evidence, presence of novel screening tests supported by evidence, or changes in the public health status of a condition. Recommendations by the USPSTF are reviewed every 5 years if no instigating factor has caused them to be assessed at an earlier time point.

When USPSTF makes a recommendation regarding a clinical preventive service, it begins establishing key research questions and commissioning a comprehensive systematic review of the literature around the topic. Although the task force weighs randomized clinical trials (level I evidence) most heavily, it does sometimes consider lower levels of evidence, such as observational studies or modeling studies. This area is one of those where politics can be injected into the task force recommendation through the inclusion or exclusion of certain types of studies based on the level of evidence. Once the systematic review of the literature is completed, the task force then meets in private, and usually does not consult disease-content experts to assist in its deliberations. The panel arrives at a draft recommendation that is then released for public comment. After the public comment period, the task force then reviews the comments and responds as it feels appropriate. It is not, however, obligated to respond to all comments. It then releases a final recommendation.

As shown in **Table 1**, the USPSTF assigns a letter grade from A to D to its recommendation regarding the particular service. Services graded an A or B are generally recommended, as there is at least a moderate certainty of net benefit. Services graded C are recommended to be selectively offered based on patient preference and/or professional judgment, owing to the likelihood of a small net benefit. Services graded D are not recommended because of a lack of net benefit, or because the benefits are outweighed by the harms. All services for which there is insufficient evidence to adequately evaluate the benefits or harms are graded an I.

The political ramifications of the USPSTF recommendations cannot be understated. Beyond the influence of the recommendations on individual patients and practitioners to commence or terminate a preventive service, the Patient Protection and Affordable Care Act (PPACA), as written, mandates full coverage with no copayment by Medicare for those preventive services that receive an A-grade or B-grade recommendation. Conversely, if a service is graded a C, D, or I, Medicare does not necessarily have to cover the service and, if it does, beneficiaries are expected to make a copayment. Obviously this has a significant impact on access to care, and may result in patients who might garner a benefit from a preventive service not receiving it.

THE USPSTF AND PROSTATE CANCER SCREENING

In May 2012, USPSTF concluded that the harms of PSA screening outweighed the potential benefits, and gave PSA screening for early detection of

Table 1 USPSTF grades for recommendations regarding clinical preventive services	
Grade	**Definition**
A	The USPSTF recommends the service. There is high certainty that the net benefit is substantial
B	The USPSTF recommends the service. There is high certainty that the net benefit is moderate, or there is moderate certainty that the net benefit is moderate to substantial
C	The USPSTF recommends selectively offering or providing this service to individual patients based on professional judgment and patient preferences. There is at least moderate certainty that the net benefit is small
D	The USPSTF recommends against the service. There is moderate or high certainty that the service has no net benefit or that the harms outweigh the benefits
I Statement	The USPSTF concludes that the current evidence is insufficient to assess the balance of benefits and harms of the service. Evidence is lacking, of poor quality, or conflicting, and the balance of benefits and harms cannot be determined

prostate cancer a grade D recommendation.[2,7,8] This recommendation was based primarily on 2 randomized clinical trials: the Prostate, Lung, Colorectal, and Ovarian (PLCO) cancer screening trial from the United States, and the European Randomized Study of Screening for Prostate Cancer (ERSPC).[2,8] Although a discussion of the strengths and weaknesses of each of these studies is beyond the scope of this article, it bears mentioning that the task force: (1) did not consider modeling studies that document a greater benefit for screening than was seen in either of the clinical trials[9]; (2) likely overestimated the mortality and other harms associated with treatment through the use of older studies[10]; and (3) did not adequately weigh the results of the strongly positive Göteborg trial[11] in its deliberations.

The larger question is: why did the Task Force handle the evidence in this manner? It is the authors' opinion that, before even starting the literature review, the Task Force had decided that it was going to recommend against prostate cancer screening. Prostate cancer care represents a significant economic burden to Medicare.[12] In addition, already overworked primary care providers really do not have the time to adequately counsel patients regarding the benefits and harms of prostate cancer screening. To this end, it would be easier and politically expeditious for the Task Force to recommend against prostate cancer screening as opposed to keeping an I recommendation or giving it a C recommendation (which would require primary care providers to spend significant amounts of time counseling men regarding PSA testing). When one considers the USPSTF's prior actions around prostate cancer screening, this argument seems to be even more valid.

Before publication of the ERSPC and PLCO trial mortality results in 2009, there was little high-quality, randomized controlled trial data with which to inform USPSTF recommendations.[2,8,13–15] That being said, the USPSTF still addressed the issue for the first time in 2002. The 2002 USPSTF report on PSA screening allowed data not only from randomized controlled trials but also from case-control studies and observational studies. Because study results were equivocal and contradictory, the Task Force concluded that there was insufficient evidence to provide a recommendation (grade I).[13,16–19]

In the 2008 report, the Task Force restricted the evidence used to inform their recommendation with regard to assessing whether a morbidity or mortality benefit existed from PSA screening.[20,21] This action would have been reasonable if there had been impactful new level I evidence on screening to inform the discussion, but at that time there were no new completed trials. Rather, the Task Force extrapolated early results from the Scandinavian Prostate Cancer Group Study 4 (SPCG-4), a trial comparing radical prostatectomy with watchful waiting, to recommend against screening for men older than 75 years (grade D).[22] Interestingly the Task Force did allow the use of cross-sectional and observational studies to inform the key question assessing the harms of PSA screening (other than overtreatment) in the 2008 report. The presumed reasoning behind the inclusion of these lower levels of evidence was that there were no clinical trials available, and none planned to explore this issue. Still, the authors contend that one could have made the same argument for the key question regarding the benefits of screening.

Because there were few such randomized controlled trials available at that time for men younger than 75, a grade I was again assigned.[14,15] The USPSTF acknowledged that they were waiting for the results of ERSPC and PLCO and, in the authors' opinion, implied in their report that unless these trials were strongly positive, the Task Force would issue a D recommendation after their release.

When the results from the ERSPC and PLCO trials were published in 2009, the USPSTF immediately began a new evidence review, which was published in 2011 ahead of the new USPSTF recommendations for PSA screening in 2012.[23] This maneuver was an unusual one that likely resulted from the backlash the USPSTF had recently received after publication of the clinical recommendations for screening mammography for early detection of breast cancer.[24] It is worth considering the USPSTF decision on prostate cancer screening in the context of the public response to the USPSTF decision on mammography and the political backlash that occurred as a consequence. Simply put, if the USPSTF had released its recommendation on prostate cancer screening concurrently with its recommendation on mammography (which likely was its original plan, given the publication date of the evidence review), it is entirely possible that there would have been congressional action to defund the USPSTF and, possibly, its parent agency AHRQ.

THE USPSTF AND BREAST CANCER SCREENING

In November 2009, the USPSTF released a recommendation statement on screening for breast cancer. Differing from common practice at that time, routine mammography for women aged 40 to 49 years was not recommended and was given a grade D recommendation, despite the confirmation of a mortality benefit in the USPSTF evidence review of screening mammography in this age group. Biennial screening mammography was recommended for women aged 50 to 74 years (grade B). The rationale for this was presumably attributable to the decreased magnitude of effectiveness of mammography screening in the younger age group (number needed to invite for screening mammography to extend one patient's life: 1904 patients for those aged 40–49 and 1339 patients for those aged 50–59).[24] It is interesting to consider how the USPSTF arrived at these estimates. The Task Force used simulation models that were developed by researchers from the CISNET breast cancer group.[25] The models assessed the cost-effectiveness of screening for breast cancer, which is surprising given that the USPSTF specifically states on their Web site that they do not consider economic costs in their decision-making process.[25] Critics of the USPSTF recommendation on breast cancer screening even contend that the Task Force did not accurately estimate the number needed to invite when they made their final recommendation.[26]

Although it is unclear whether this is definitively the case, there is certainly some merit to the claim and it begs several questions. First, why is the USPSTF using cost-effectiveness models when it explicitly states it is not going to consider cost; second, are their estimates of effect accurate; and third, why are they even using models in the first place if they state that they only will allow level I evidence to document a benefit? Their own meta-analysis of the trials for mammography in women aged 40 to 49 documents that there is a benefit, so it seems that additional modeling would only be needed if the results of the meta-analysis did not fit with the Task Force's political agenda. Of note, there are similar models for prostate cancer screening that document a benefit,[27] but in the case of PSA screening the USPSTF established a different set of rules for reasons unclear.

Regardless, the outcry from professional organizations, patient advocacy groups, the media, and the public at large to the mammography decision was strident and defiant. Elected officials were pushed into action and indeed, Secretary Sebelius of the Department of Health and Human Services advised that screening mammography continue to start at age 40 years. Within a month, the USPSTF altered the language of the recommendation for women aged 40 to 49 to reflect the individual nature of the decision to undergo screening mammography without recommending against screening (but maintained a grade D recommendation).

Unfortunately, there was no similar public outcry with the release of the prostate cancer recommendations. Although the American Urological Association (AUA) expressed "outrage" at the decision, this carried little weight, presumably because, as specialists who may stand to gain professionally and financially from prostate cancer screening, we are viewed as irreversibly biased. Had there been a strong response from the patient advocacy community and the media, however, things might have been different, as these stakeholders have considerably more political clout. Unfortunately, although there was pushback from the patient advocacy groups it was somewhat muted compared with the response to the mammography decision, and ultimately it had little effect.

POLITICAL NEXT STEPS IN THE PROSTATE CANCER SCREENING DEBATE

The discussion around prostate cancer screening is far from over. Since the release of the USPSTF recommendation, numerous other organizations have issued guidelines on the topic. The American College of Physicians,[28] The European Association of Urology,[29] the National Comprehensive Cancer Center Coalition,[30] and the AUA[31] have all issued guidelines that endorse informed decision making around prostate cancer screening, in direct contrast to the USPSTF recommendation. The new AUA guidelines, in particular, have important political ramifications in the debate. Specifically, the guidelines do not recommend routine PSA screening in men at average risk for prostate cancer ages 40 to 55 years, which is a change from the 2009 AUA best practice panel statement. This updated statement, which does not specifically recommend against prostate cancer screening but is evidence based and acknowledges that the clinical trials do not support population-wide screening in this setting, helps reestablish urology's credibility in the debate. Similarly, the guidelines do not recommend screening in men older than 70, which is in line with the evidence and with other organizations' recommendations. Importantly the guidelines specifically discourage mass screening events, such as testing at health fairs, where shared decision making is unlikely to occur.

A second key political initiative is to encourage the USPSTF to review its decision using existing mechanisms. The USPSTF reviews its recommendations at regular intervals, when new evidence becomes available and when there are enough public stakeholder requests. Interested parties are encouraged to go to the USPSTF Web site (available at: http://www.uspreventiveservices taskforce.org/tftopicnon.htm) and submit an electronic request to review the recommendation on prostate cancer screening.

Finally, efforts are currently under way to improve the efficiency and transparency of the USPSTF in the form of the USPSTF Transparency and Accountability Act of 2013 (HR 2143, https://www.govtrack.us/congress/bills/113/hr2143), introduced by Marsha Blackburn (R-Tn), which has bipartisan support. This bill also includes provisions for decreasing the USPSTF impact in the PPACA and for increased inclusion of specialists, and also is endorsed by the AUA. The Act is a key priority on the AUA's legislative agenda, and is having an effect. Specifically, the USPSTF and AHRQ have already volunteered to incorporate some of the recommendations in the bill into the process, potentially obviating the legislation. While the changes that have been made are promising they are by no means adequate, and there is still a need for this legislation.

SUMMARY

It is of particular importance that urologists have a voice in the creation of health policy for conditions that we directly diagnose and treat. Although there is no danger yet for denial of coverage of PSA screening by Medicare, it will be important to urge the USPSTF to review their recommendation against PSA screening for men of all ages so that well-informed patients who might potentially benefit from the early detection of prostate cancer by PSA screening can continue to do so. Urologists must become more politically active on this issue in an effort to advance the health of their patients and reduce the public health burden of prostate cancer in the United States.

REFERENCES

1. Koss LG. The Papanicolaou test for cervical cancer detection. A triumph and a tragedy. JAMA 1989; 261:737.
2. Schroder FH, Hugosson J, Roobol MJ, et al. Screening and prostate-cancer mortality in a randomized European study. N Engl J Med 2009;360:1320.
3. National comprehensive cancer network guidelines and derivative information products: user guide. 2013. Available at: http://www.nccn.org/clinical.asp. Accessed February 12, 2014.
4. Heidenreich A, Bastian PJ, Bellmunt J, et al. EAU guidelines on prostate cancer. part 1: screening, diagnosis, and local treatment with curative intent-update 2013. Eur Urol 2014;65(1):124–37.
5. USPSTF: About the United States Preventive Services Task Force. Rockville (MD); 2013. Available at: http://www.uspreventiveservicestaskforce.org/about.htm. Accessed February 12, 2014.
6. Brawley O, Byers T, Chen A, et al. New American Cancer Society process for creating trustworthy cancer screening guidelines. JAMA 2011;306:2495.
7. Moyer VA. Screening for prostate cancer: U.S. Preventive Services Task Force recommendation statement. Ann Intern Med 2012;157:120.
8. Andriole GL, Crawford ED, Grubb RL 3rd, et al. Mortality results from a randomized prostate-cancer screening trial. N Engl J Med 2009;360:1310.
9. Etzioni R, Gulati R, Cooperberg MR, et al. Limitations of basing screening policies on screening trials: the US Preventive Services Task Force and Prostate Cancer Screening. Med Care 2013;51:295.
10. Yao SL, Lu-Yao G. Population-based study of relationships between hospital volume of prostatectomies,

11. Hugosson J, Carlsson S, Aus G, et al. Mortality results from the Goteborg randomised population-based prostate-cancer screening trial. Lancet Oncol 2010;11:725.
12. Penson DF, Chan JM. Prostate cancer. J Urol 2007; 177:2020.
13. Labrie F, Candas B, Dupont A, et al. Screening decreases prostate cancer death: first analysis of the 1988 Quebec prospective randomized controlled trial. Prostate 1999;38:83.
14. Labrie F, Candas B, Cusan L, et al. Screening decreases prostate cancer mortality: 11-year follow-up of the 1988 Quebec prospective randomized controlled trial. Prostate 2004;59:311.
15. Sandblom G, Varenhorst E, Lofman O, et al. Clinical consequences of screening for prostate cancer: 15 years follow-up of a randomised controlled trial in Sweden. Eur Urol 2004;46:717.
16. U.S. Preventive Services Task Force. Screening for prostate cancer: recommendation and rationale. Ann Intern Med 2002;137:915.
17. Harris R, Lohr KN. Screening for prostate cancer: an update of the evidence for the U.S. Preventive Services Task Force. Ann Intern Med 2002;137:917.
18. Jacobsen SJ, Bergstralh EJ, Katusic SK, et al. Screening digital rectal examination and prostate cancer mortality: a population-based case-control study. Urology 1998;52:173.
19. Richert-Boe KE, Humphrey LL, Glass AG, et al. Screening digital rectal examination and prostate cancer mortality: a case-control study. J Med Screen 1998;5:99.
20. U.S. Preventive Services Task Force. Screening for prostate cancer: U.S. Preventive Services Task Force recommendation statement. Ann Intern Med 2008;149:185.
21. Lin K, Lipsitz R, Miller T, et al. Benefits and harms of prostate-specific antigen screening for prostate cancer: an evidence update for the U.S. Preventive Services Task Force. Ann Intern Med 2008;149:192.
22. Bill-Axelson A, Holmberg L, Ruutu M, et al. Radical prostatectomy versus watchful waiting in early prostate cancer. N Engl J Med 2005;352:1977.
23. Chou R, Croswell JM, Dana T, et al. Screening for prostate cancer: a review of the evidence for the U.S. Preventive Services Task Force. Ann Intern Med 2011;155:762.
24. US Preventive Services Task Force. Screening for breast cancer: U.S. Preventive Services Task Force recommendation statement. Ann Intern Med 2009; 151:716.
25. Mandelblatt JS, Cronin KA, Bailey S, et al. Effects of mammography screening under different screening schedules: model estimates of potential benefits and harms. Ann Intern Med 2009;151:738.

26. Hendrick RE, Helvie MA. Mammography screening: a new estimate of number needed to screen to prevent one breast cancer death. AJR Am J Roentgenol 2012;198:723.

27. Etzioni R, Tsodikov A, Mariotto A, et al. Quantifying the role of PSA screening in the US prostate cancer mortality decline. Cancer Causes Control 2008;19:175.

28. Qaseem A, Barry MJ, Denberg TD, et al. Screening for prostate cancer: a guidance statement from the Clinical Guidelines Committee of the American College of Physicians. Ann Intern Med 2013;158:761.

29. Heidenreich A, Abrahamsson PA, Artibani W, et al. Early detection of prostate cancer: European Association of Urology recommendation. Eur Urol 2013; 64(3):347–54.

30. National Comprehensive Cancer Network: prostate cancer early detection. 2012. Available at: http://www.nccn.org/professionals/physician_gls/pdf/prostate_detection.pdf. Accessed February 12, 2014.

31. Carter HB, Albertsen PC, Barry MJ, et al. Early detection of prostate cancer: AUA guideline. J Urol 2013;190:419.

Decision Making and Prostate Cancer Screening

Sara J. Knight, PhD[a,b,c],*

KEYWORDS

- Prostate cancer screening • Prostate specific antigen (PSA) test • Informed decision making
- Shared decision making • Patient decision aid • Patient preferences • Patient values
- Values clarification

KEY POINTS

- Prostate cancer screening is a significant decision for men because of the concerns about survival with prostate cancer and the downstream impacts of biopsy and treatment that may impact many years of a man's life.
- Prostate cancer screening is widely regarded as a preference-sensitive decision for men where the importance that a man places on the benefits and harms of screening and treatment is seen as central to choice of screening.
- Prostate cancer screening decisions are complex and challenging for men because of affective and cognitive factors, such as anxiety about cancer and the tendency to rely on personal experience and anecdotes about screening over scientific evidence.
- Guideline recommendations for prostate cancer screening emphasize a shared decision-making approach that involves collaboration between a man and his health professionals.
- Patient decision aids have been designed for prostate cancer screening with the aim of improving decision quality, increasing the alignment between a man's values, goals, and preferences with the ultimate choice, and reducing necessary practice variation.

Prostate cancer screening decisions are important to men and their families, involving significant consequences that will potentially influence many years of a man's life. Currently, screening for prostate cancer is surrounded by more controversy than many other health decisions. Although prostate cancer screening using prostate-specific antigen (PSA) testing has been used since the 1980s for early detection of prostate cancer with associated declines in prostate cancer mortality, concern about harms of PSA screening has been raised, including the potential for false-positive results leading to unnecessary biopsies and the risk of pain and infection. There is also the potential for overtreatment of indolent prostate cancer that would be unlikely to progress during a man's lifetime. The adverse consequences of surgical and radiation treatment for prostate cancer have been well documented, including pain, incontinence, sexual dysfunction, and bowel problems. The benefit from prostate cancer screening has been questioned, particularly for men older than 74, especially in those who have comorbidities and life expectancy is less than 10 years.[1–3]

Disclosures Funding Sources: None.
Disclosures Conflict of Interest: None.
[a] Health Services Research and Development Service, Office of Research and Development, Veterans Health Administration, 810 Vermont Avenue, Northwest, Washington, DC 20420, USA; [b] Department of Psychiatry, University of California San Francisco, 401 Parnassus Avenue, San Francisco, CA 94143, USA; [c] Department of Urology, University of California San Francisco, 400 Parnassus Avenue, Suite A610, San Francisco, CA 94123, USA
* Health Services Research and Development Service, Office of Research and Development, Veterans Health Administration, 810 Vermont Avenue, Northwest, Washington, DC 20420.
E-mail address: sara.knight@va.gov

Urol Clin N Am 41 (2014) 257–266
http://dx.doi.org/10.1016/j.ucl.2014.01.008
0094-0143/14/$ – see front matter Published by Elsevier Inc.

Despite two large randomized trials and several meta-analyses on the early detection of prostate cancer a lack of clarity remains for many men.[4–7] Based on this evidence, the US Preventive Services Task Force (USPSTF) does not recommend routine prostate cancer screening using PSA testing in men of any age.[8] However, criticism of how the USPSTF has interpreted the evidence has been raised.[9] Other professional and scientific organizations have developed alternate guidelines.[10–14] Recognizing the importance of the decision to men and questions about the value of screening has led professional and scientific societies to recommend that decisions about prostate cancer screening using PSA testing be based on informed decision making with consideration of the potential benefits and harms and the alternatives to screening.

This article considers decisions about prostate cancer screening, highlighting the challenges that these choices present for men, their families, and their health care professionals, including complex emotions and cognitive factors, and conflicting guideline recommendations. Shared decision making is considered as an approach to helping men make these choices, and resources, such as patient decision aids, are discussed.

WHY ARE PROSTATE CANCER SCREENING DECISIONS SO CHALLENGING?

Aside from the confusion created by conflicting guideline recommendations, prostate cancer screening decisions are emotionally and cognitively complicated. False-positive prostate cancer screening results have been associated with persistent psychological distress, even with a negative biopsy.[15] High anxiety in men with a family history of prostate cancer has been associated with increased use of prostate cancer screening,[16] and among men who had visited doctors frequently, anxiety was associated with increased PSA testing.[17]

In addition to affect, Arkes and Gaissmaier[18] point to several cognitive factors that further complicate prostate cancer screening decisions. For example, anecdotal evidence and personal experience can be persuasive even in light of contradictory data. Even when data are available, the interpretation may be challenging due to tendencies to disregard contextual information such as base rates.

WHAT DO PROSTATE CANCER SCREENING GUIDELINES SAY ABOUT DECISION MAKING?

In many difficult health care choices, guidelines offer patients and health professionals clear pathways for care that are based on evidence, consensus of experts, or best practices. Guidelines have recommended PSA screening as a population-based approach for the early detection of prostate cancer with the goal of reducing mortality from prostate cancer, and observational studies have shown a decrease in mortality starting in the 1990s when PSA testing was widely used.[19] During the past decade, guidelines for prostate cancer screening have been revised to reflect evidence that PSA testing for prostate cancer is associated with significant harms related to overtesting and overtreatment of low-risk disease.

Current guidelines have been developed and disseminated by federal agencies, foundations, and professional and scientific societies, and there are considerable differences among guideline developers in the interpretation of the evidence and its implications for policy and clinical practice.[8,10–14] **Table 1** summarizes 6 of the current guidelines for screening or early detection of prostate cancer. None of these guidelines recommends universal screening for prostate cancer using PSA or any other available method. The USPSTF presents the most limited use of screening, discouraging PSA screening for men of any age and suggests that informed decision making be used only when men request a PSA test.[8] In contrast, the American Cancer Society (ACS) recommends that average-risk men be screened for prostate cancer using PSA testing starting at age 50 if the man is informed about the alternatives to testing, the potential benefits, and the risk of harms. The ACS guideline encourages testing at younger ages for men at higher than average risk, including African American men, for whom the ACS recommends screening starting at age 45, and those with a family history of prostate cancer for whom the ACS recommends screening starting at age 40. The ACS guideline endorses informing men about the benefits and harms of early detection and treatment and considering a man's values, goals, and preferences about using PSA testing for early detection.[14]

Many contemporary guidelines encourage a shared decision-making approach to prostate cancer screening. Shared decision making typically involves communication between patient and health professional, where information is shared about the options in the choice (eg, to screen or not) and the expected outcomes of each option (eg, survival, side effects with treatment, anxiety, late detection of prostate cancer), including the scientific uncertainty surrounding the expected benefits and harms.[20–22] Downstream consequences of the choice alternatives also may be described in shared decision making, such as the risk of having repeated biopsies and the potential for diagnosis of low-risk prostate cancer that is unlikely to contribute to mortality, but that is frequently treated once found.[3,23] In addition to information, shared decision making also involves the man and his health professional coming to an understanding of the man's values, goals, and preferences relevant to the options and where the trade-offs between the benefits and harms are considered from the patient's perspective.[21,22,24]

Although many guidelines are specific about using shared decision making, others emphasize an informed decision-making approach in which the emphasis is placed on providing information and less on understanding the patient's values, goals, and preferences relevant to the choice.[25] All of the guidelines shown in **Table 1** suggest the use of either shared or informed decision making, but they differ in when and how informed or shared decision making should be implemented. The USPSTF recommendations stand out as focusing primarily on providing information to those men who request screening an approach that would engage only a highly select group of men in an informed decision making process. The USPSTF recommendations do not include explicit consideration of a man's values, goals, and preferences relevant to screening.[8] Other guidelines favor some degree of shared decision making. For example, the American College of Preventive Medicine recommends no routine screening at any age, but suggests that all men be informed about the potential risks and benefits of prostate cancer screening and that the man's preferences be considered in the final choice.[12] The ACS, American College of Physicians, American Society of Clinical Oncology (ASCO), and American Urology Association (AUA) recommend that men be informed about the risks and benefits of screening.[10,11,13,14] ASCO and the AUA guidelines explicitly recommend a shared decision-making approach in which the information exchange occurs in the context of a discussion between a man and his health professionals.[10,11]

Screening for prostate cancer has been considered to be a preference-sensitive decision in which several reasonable choice alternatives are available (eg, screening vs no screening) that differ in terms of their characteristics and outcomes (eg, potential benefits and harms) (**Box 1**).[24,26] How a man values the potential benefits and harms is considered to be central to a preference-sensitive decision when there is clearly more than one effective option available. O'Connor and colleagues[24] have differentiated between "preference-sensitive

decisions" when there is no difference in effectiveness between several options and "effective decisions" when evidence is available to support the effectiveness of one option. In "effective decisions," the goal is uptake of the effective option, or in the case of prostate cancer screening, the goal would be implementation of smarter screening based on prostate cancer risk characteristics.

Many of the guidelines in **Table 1** emphasize consideration of a man's preferences for screening. The ACS guidelines discuss preferences explicitly and recommend that screening be offered if consistent with a man's preferences.[14] ASCO guidelines consider preferences implicitly recommending an individualized approach to PSA testing based on a discussion of the potential harms and benefits of potentially unnecessary tests and treatments.[10] The AUA guidelines place an emphasis on preferences referring to a man's values, goals, and preferences for screening as a central consideration in PSA testing.[11]

IMPLEMENTATION OF SCREENING GUIDELINES

The public response to the revised guidelines suggests that many men do not embrace recommendations to limit PSA testing and screening for prostate cancer. Most of these surveys of the implementation prostate cancer screening guidelines have focused on the USPSTF recommendations. For example, Caire and colleagues[27] found that most of those men seen in a screening clinic disagreed with the earlier USPSTF recommendations to discontinue screening at age 75. More recently, a survey of a national online panel found that 62% agreed with USPSTF recommendations against prostate cancer screening with PSA, but only 13% intended to follow the guidelines and forego PSA testing.[28] Those who were more worried about prostate cancer and older men were more likely to disagree with the USPSTF guidelines and those of African American race and those with higher incomes, with greater worry about prostate cancer, and with prior use of PSA testing were more likely to have PSA testing.[28] The 2010 National Health Interview Survey results are consistent with limited use of PSA testing for prostate cancer with almost one-half (44.2%) reporting that they have not had prior PSA testing to screen for prostate cancer.[26]

Adoption of the USPSTF recommendations among primary care providers has been modest. PSA screening practices decreased slightly following the introduction of the USPSTF recommendations against screening men older than 74

Table 1
Prostate cancer screening guidelines and recommendations

Author	Year	Population	Recommendation		
			Screening or Early Detection for Average-Risk Men	Informed Decision Making[2]	Patient Preferences Considered[3]
ACS	2013	• Start PSA testing at 50 y for all • Start PSA testing at 45 y for African Americans • Start PSA testing at 40 y for men with first-degree relatives diagnosed with prostate cancer	Recommends PSA for early detection starting at age 50 for average-risk men if patient is informed and if consistent with preferences	Yes	Yes

ACP	2013	• No screening for any age if the man's preferences are not to screen
		• Start screening between age 50 and 69 if
		  ○ Life expectancy of at least 10 y
		  ○ Information has been provided on the limited potential for benefits and substantial risk of harm associated with prostate cancer screening
		  ○ Consistent with preferences
			Recommends no screening of average-risk men younger than 50, older than 69, or those with a life expectancy of less than 10–15 y
			Clinicians consider the following in their recommendations for screening: risk for prostate cancer, discussion of the benefits and harms of screening, consideration of the man's general health and comorbid conditions, life expectancy, and preferences
				Yes	Yes

ACPM	2008	• No general screening in any men with either digital rectal examination or with PSA • Those at high risk, including African Americans and men with a family history of prostate cancer may benefit from screening	Recommends no screening at any age and that men should be given information about the potential benefits and harms of screening and the limits of current evidence	Yes	Yes
ASCO	2012	• No general screening in men with life expectancy of 10 y or less • Screening in men with life expectancy of more than 10 y after discussion of potential benefits and harms	Recommends individualized screening based life expectancy and after discussion of benefits and harms, including complications from unnecessary diagnostic tests or treatments	Yes, using lay language	Not discussed explicitly

(continued on next page)

and those with life expectancy fewer than 10 to 15 years. Following the USPSTF recommendations in 2008, PSA testing in men older than 75 years cared for in the Veterans Health Administration declined slightly, and additional small declines in PSA testing of 3.0% and 2.7% among those 40 to 54 years of age and 55 to 74 years of age, respectively, were observed

Table 1
(continued)

Author	Year	Population	Recommendation		
			Screening or Early Detection for Average-Risk Men	Informed Decision Making[2]	Patient Preferences Considered[3]
AUA	2013	• No screening age 54 or younger • Shared decision making and screening only when based on men's values and goals for age 55–69 y • No screening for age 70 or older, or life expectancy less than 10 y	Recommends shared decision making for early detection based on men's values and goals between 55 and 69 y; no screening if life expectancy is less than 10 y for any age older than 54	Yes	Yes, values and preferences are a central consideration
USPSTF	2011	• No screening at any age for all men	Does not recommend screening for prostate cancer using PSA testing for any age or population; recommends providing information about the screening alternatives, potential benefits, and risk of harms, if a man requests screening	Yes, if a man requests screening	Not discussed explicitly

Abbreviations: ACP, American College of Physicians; ACPM, American College of Preventive Medicine; ACS, American Cancer Society; ASCO, American Society of Clinical Oncology; AUA, American Urology Association; PSA, prostate-specific antigen; USPSTF, US Preventive Services Task Force.

following these publications in 2009.[29] Among 89 primary care providers responding to a national Internet survey in 2010, 51% and 64% indicated that they discuss and order PSA testing for men between 50 and 74, respectively. Only 21% and 28% indicated that their screening practices had been influenced by the 2009 publications of the European Randomized Screening for Prostate Cancer and the Prostate, Lung, Colorectal and Ovarian trials, respectively.[30] Others observed a small, but significant, decrease in PSA testing (8.6% vs 7.6%) following publication of the 2011 USPSTF recommendations against screening in all men regardless of age or life expectancy.[31] Although almost half of primary care providers (49.2%) in a health care system said that they agreed with the 2011 USPSTF recommendations against universal screening, many fewer (1.8%) said that they would no longer order PSA testing for their patients and 37.7% said that they would not change their PSA testing practice based on the USPSTF guidelines. Providers cited several barriers to stopping PSA testing in their patients who had previously participated in prostate cancer screening, including patient expectations of screening, lack of time to discuss changes in recommendations, worry about malpractice litigation, and discomfort with uncertainty.[32]

In addition to recommending that prostate cancer screening using PSA testing be based on age and other clinical risk factors, all guidelines with

Box 1
Preference-sensitive decision characteristics

• Several choice alternatives in which one is not clearly better than the other(s) and each is associated with unique characteristics and expected outcomes

• Decision-maker's values and preferences for the choice alternative characteristics and expected outcomes are considered to be important determinants of the choice

• In making the decision, information about the alternatives and their characteristics is considered; values, goals, and preferences for the alternatives are identified and compared; a choice is made based on the value of the alternatives to the individual making the choice

the exception of those of the USPSTF guidelines recommend shared decision making and that the choice of screening be based on the man's preferences. The types of shared decision making suggested by the guidelines include (1) providing information on the alternatives for prostate cancer screening, potential benefits and harms, and uncertainties associated with the various outcomes, and (2) assessing the man's preferences for screening alternatives (eg, PSA testing vs no PSA testing) or for the potential outcomes and downstream impacts of screening (eg, survival, false-positive rate, anxiety associated with prostate cancer, treatment and its associated impacts on urinary and sexual function).

In contrast to guideline recommendations, studies of informed decision making in prostate cancer screening has suggested that many men receive PSA testing without being fully informed.[26,33,34] A recent nationally representative sample of men between ages 49 and 75 responding to the National Health Interview Survey reported that most (64.3%) had not had any previous discussions with their physicians about PSA screening and its benefits and harms and associated uncertainties, and only 8% of the respondents reported discussion of 3 key elements of shared decision making (ie, advantages, disadvantages, and scientific uncertainties). The absence of shared decision making was associated with no screening rather than with screening.[26]

SHARED DECISION MAKING AND PATIENT DECISION AIDS

Shared decision making is a central principle embodied in the Institute of Medicine concept of patient-centered care, including decisions about screening.[35] Patient decision aids are decision support technologies that have been developed to support shared decision making, to improve the quality of the decision, and to reduce variation in care and unnecessary tests and treatment (**Box 2**). Most patient decision aids aim to increase knowledge necessary to make an informed decision and to improve the agreement between a patient's values, goals, and preferences and the choice.[24] Distinct from patient education materials, patient decision aids aim to provide information that is based on the considerations and concerns that patients have in making the decision and that is balanced and free from bias.[24] In addition to information, patient decision aids include methods to help patients identify what is most important to them in considering the characteristics of the alternatives, including the outcomes. Many decision aids provide value

---

> **Box 2**
> **Key elements of patient decision aids**
>
> - Balanced information on the condition, the decision, the choice alternatives, the characteristics and outcomes of each alternative, and the scientific uncertainty associated with the outcomes
> - Tools that assist with the identification and clarification of values, goals, and preferences relevant to the decision, the choice alternatives, and the outcomes
> - Guidance in deliberation that will assist with the comparison of the alternatives, weighing of the values and goals, and considering the trade-offs in values and goals that may be needed to make the choice
> - Coaching in communication of values and goals to family members and health professionals
> - Disclosure of any potential bias or conflict of interest in the development and presentation of the decision aid
> - Systematic development of the patient decision aid that includes the following:
>   - Input from patients with the condition or health concern and health professionals and other experts
>   - Field testing in clinical and community settings
>   - Evaluation of the decision aid

---

clarification exercises and other tools that support deliberation and consideration of the trade-offs in values and goals that may be needed in making the choice. Finally, some decision aids provide coaching or guidance in communication of values, goals, and preferences to their family members and health professionals.[36]

Decision aid development efforts have focused attention on prostate cancer screening choices and a number of tools are available currently. Seven online decision aids are shown in **Table 2** to illustrate the breadth of format and features. Decision aids are available in print, in electronic media, and online. The decision aids provided by the ACS, ASCO, and the Centers for Disease Control and Prevention are available online in pdf files. They are written in plain language and are brief and easy to download. Some decision aids that are interactive, such as those provided by Healthwise and Healthdialog, and can be individualized according to clinical risk factors and values, goals, and preferences. Many decision aids include

Table 2	
Decision aids for patients prostate cancer screening and early detection	
Development Organization/Host[a]	**Decision Aid**
American Cancer Society	http://www.cancer.org/acs/groups/content/@editorial/documents/document/acspc-024618.pdf
American Society of Clinical Oncology	http://stage.asco.org/sites/default/files/psa_pco_decision_aid_71612.pdf
Centers for Disease Control and Prevention	http://www.uspreventiveservicestaskforce.org/prostatecancerscreening/prostatecancerfact.pdf
Informed Medical Decisions Foundation/ Health Dialogue/Healthcrossroads	https://www.healthcrossroads.com/example/crossroad.aspx?contentGUID=fc326615-5b29-47f1-87c3-9a3e2d946919
Healthwise/Intermountain Healthcare	http://intermountainhealthcare.org/health-resources/health-topics/healthwise/content/aa38144/prostate-cancer-screening-should-i-have-a-psa-test.aspx#zx3721
Mayo Clinic	http://www.mayoclinic.com/health/prostate-cancer/HQ01273
National Cancer Institute	http://www.cancer.gov/cancertopics/factsheet/Detection/PSA

[a] Organization responsible for development of the decision aid/host of online decision aid when different from the development organization.

pictographs depicting risk information graphically, as well as numerically and in text. Some decision aids include videos of patients who share their experiences making prostate cancer screening decisions or who talk about how they managed the side effects from biopsy or treatment.

The International Patient Decision Aids Standards (IPDAS) Collaboration, a multiple stakeholder initiative including scientists, clinicians, patients, and representatives from health plans, developed a set of standards for the development and dissemination of decision support tools for patients.[36,37] The collaboration used a systematic Delphi process and conducted additional studies to refine and validate the standards. Members of the collaboration have developed a measure to evaluate the quality of decision aids. The IPDAS instrument (IPDASi) has incorporated 10 domains and 47 items. IPDASi domains and example item themes are listed in **Table 3**.[36,37] The domains include (1) the types of information that should be included for treatments and tests with an emphasis on the balance of information, including both positive and negative characteristics of the choice alternatives; (2) methods including comparisons of the choice alternatives that will assist in the identification and expression of values that are relevant to the decision; (3) guidance on how to deliberate in a systematic way to facilitate weighing the decision alternatives according to one's values; (4) criteria that are critical to the process of developing the decision aid, such as

patient and expert input; and (5) elements that are needed to evaluate the tool.

A recent Cochrane Collaboration review suggested that decision aids for treatment and screening decisions improved patient and health professional communication, increased patient engagement, and improved knowledge, but had a mixed effect on the length of consultation and the actual choices. In addition, those decision aids that offered tools and methods to explicitly elicit and clarify patient values improved choices that were consistent with the values.[38] A review of prostate cancer screening decision aids found that, in 18 primary care and community-based studies, decision aids increased patient knowledge and confidence and reduced decision conflict.[39] Although the decision aids had no effect on screening behavior of those seeking screening services, they contributed to a decrease in interest in PSA testing among those seeking routine care.[39] Similarly, studies published since this review have found variable results for choice of PSA testing, with some showing higher levels of PSA testing[40] and others showing lower levels.[41] These and other decision aids differ widely in methods, such as level of information and balance in presentation, potentially contributing to variation in findings across studies of decision aids.

As interest in patient decision aids has expanded, so have efforts to understand and measure patient preferences, and innovative work on

Table 3
International Patient Decision Aid Standards instrument domains and example item themes

Domains	Example Item Themes
Information	• Describes the health condition or problem • Describes the options available • Shows the negative and positive features of options with equal detail
Probabilities	• Provides information about outcome probabilities associated with the options • Specifies the defined group for the outcome probabilities • Allows comparison of the outcome probabilities across the options
Values	• Describes the features of options to help patients imagine what it is like to experience the physical effects • Asks patients to think about which positive and negative features of the options matter most to them
Decision guidance	• Provides a step-by-step way to make a decision • Includes tools like worksheets or lists of questions to use when discussing options
Development	• Process included identification of what patients need to prepare them to discuss a specific decision • Process included expert review by patients and health professionals • Process included field testing with patients and health professionals
Evidence	• Describes how research evidence was selected or synthesized • Provides citations to the studies selected • Describes the quality of the evidence used
Disclosure	• Provides information about the funding used for development
Plain language	• Reports readability levels of the information presented
Decision support technology evaluation	• Process included accumulation of evidence that the decision support technology improves the match between patient values, goals, and preferences and the choice
Test (for those decision support technologies focused on screening tests)	• Describes what the test is designed to measure • Includes information about the chances of having true or false positive and negative test results • Describes the next steps if the test detects the condition or if the condition is not detected

values has contributed several new instruments.[42] Despite a large number of clinical trials, there has been little implementation of decision aids in clinical or community settings.[43,44] Arterburn and colleagues at Group Health Research have moved in this direction with their study of 12 decision aids in an integrated health care system.[45] Although this work did not include prostate cancer screening decisions, several recent studies on prostate cancer screening decisions have conducted pre-implementation studies in men of lower income and education levels in community settings.[46,47]

SUMMARY

Prostate cancer screening decisions are significant to men and their families, considering the potential for benefits, including survival and the possibility of harms from overtesting and overtreatment that can impact a man's life for many years. These decisions are challenging because of emotions associated with prostate cancer, as well as common cognitive tendencies, such as weighing personal experience with a prostate cancer survivor more heavily than research data on the benefits and harms of PSA testing. In addition, scientific and professional organizations have taken disparate interpretations of the research evidence on the effectiveness of PSA screening for prostate cancer; consequently, recommendations for prostate cancer screening differ across guidelines. Current guidelines are in agreement, however, on the importance of taking an informed decision-making or a shared decision-making approach to prostate cancer screening. Informed or shared decision making endorses providing patients with information on the potential benefits and harms associated with screening and considering what is important to a patient in evaluating the benefits and harms. Patient decision aids have been developed to assist in this process, with outcomes including improved knowledge, realistic perceptions of the benefits and harms, lower decision conflict, and improved agreement between the man's values and his choices about screening.

REFERENCES

1. Kotwal AA, Mohile SG, Dale W. Remaining life expectancy measurement and PSA screening of older men. J Geriatr Oncol 2012;3(3):196–204.

2. Walter LC, Bertenthal D, Lindquist K, et al. PSA screening among elderly men with limited life expectancies. JAMA 2006;296(19):2336–42.

3. Walter LC, Fung KZ, Kirby KA, et al. Five-year downstream outcomes following prostate-specific antigen screening in older men. JAMA Intern Med 2013; 173(10):866–73.

4. Andriole GL, Crawford ED, Grubb RL 3rd, et al. Mortality results from a randomized prostate-cancer screening trial. N Engl J Med 2009;360(13):1310–9.

5. Djulbegovic M, Beyth RJ, Neuberger MM, et al. Screening for prostate cancer: systematic review and meta-analysis of randomised controlled trials. BMJ 2010;341:c4543.

6. Ilic D, Neuberger MM, Djulbegovic M, et al. Screening for prostate cancer. Cochrane Database Syst Rev 2013;(1):CD004720.

7. Schroder FH, Hugosson J, Roobol MJ, et al. Screening and prostate-cancer mortality in a randomized European study. N Engl J Med 2009;360(13): 1320–8.

8. Moyer VA. Screening for prostate cancer: U.S. Preventive Services Task Force recommendation statement. Ann Intern Med 2012;157(2):120–34.

9. Etzioni R, Gulati R, Cooperberg MR, et al. Limitations of basing screening policies on screening trials: the US preventive services task force and prostate cancer screening. Med Care 2013;51(4): 295–300.

10. Basch E, Oliver TK, Vickers A, et al. Screening for prostate cancer with prostate-specific antigen testing: American Society of Clinical Oncology Provisional Clinical Opinion. J Clin Oncol 2012;30(24): 3020–5.

11. Carter HB, Albertsen PC, Barry MJ, et al. Early detection of prostate cancer: AUA Guideline. J Urol 2013;190(2):419–26.

12. Lim LS, Sherin K. Screening for prostate cancer in US men ACPM position statement on preventive practice. Am J Prev Med 2008;34(2):164–70.

13. Qaseem A, Barry MJ, Denberg TD, et al. Screening for prostate cancer: a guidance statement from the Clinical Guidelines Committee of the American College of Physicians. Ann Intern Med 2013;158(10): 761–9.

14. Wolf AM, Wender RC, Etzioni RB, et al. American Cancer Society guideline for the early detection of prostate cancer: update 2010. CA Cancer J Clin 2010;60(2):70–98.

15. Katz DA, Jarrard DF, McHorney CA, et al. Health perceptions in patients who undergo screening and workup for prostate cancer. Urology 2007; 69(2):215–20.

16. Taylor KL, Shelby R, Kerner J, et al. Impact of undergoing prostate carcinoma screening on prostate carcinoma-related knowledge and distress. Cancer 2002;95(5):1037–44.

17. Kotwal AA, Schumm P, Mohile SG, et al. The influence of stress, depression, and anxiety on PSA screening rates in a nationally representative sample. Med Care 2012;50(12):1037–44.

18. Arkes HR, Gaissmaier W. Psychological research and the prostate-cancer screening controversy. Psychol Sci 2012;23(6):547–53.

19. Greene KL, Albertsen PC, Babaian RJ, et al. Prostate specific antigen best practice statement: 2009 update. J Urol 2013;189(Suppl 1):S2–11.

20. Cribb A, Entwistle VA. Shared decision making: trade-offs between narrower and broader conceptions. Health Expect 2011;14(2):210–9.

21. Moumjid N, Gafni A, Bremond A, et al. Shared decision making in the medical encounter: are we all talking about the same thing? Med Decis Making 2007;27(5):539–46.

22. O'Connor AM, Llewellyn-Thomas HA, Flood AB. Modifying unwarranted variations in health care: shared decision making using patient decision aids. Health Aff (Millwood) 2004;(Suppl Variation): VAR63–72.

23. Zeliadt SB, Hoffman RM, Etzioni R, et al. What happens after an elevated PSA test: the experience of 13,591 veterans. J Gen Intern Med 2010;25(11): 1205–10.

24. O'Connor AM, Wennberg JE, Legare F, et al. Toward the 'tipping point': decision aids and informed patient choice. Health Aff (Millwood) 2007;26(3): 716–25.

25. Rimer BK, Briss PA, Zeller PK, et al. Informed decision making: what is its role in cancer screening? Cancer 2004;101(Suppl 5):1214–28.

26. Han PK, Kobrin S, Breen N, et al. National evidence on the use of shared decision making in prostate-specific antigen screening. Ann Fam Med 2013; 11(4):306–14.

27. Caire AA, Sun L, Robertson CN, et al. Public survey and survival data do not support recommendations to discontinue prostate-specific antigen screening in men at age 75. Urology 2010;75(5):1122–7.

28. Squiers LB, Bann CM, Dolina SE, et al. Prostate-specific antigen testing: men's responses to 2012 recommendation against screening. Am J Prev Med 2013;45(2):182–9.

29. Zeliadt SB, Hoffman RM, Etzioni R, et al. Influence of publication of US and European prostate cancer screening trials on PSA testing practices. J Natl Cancer Inst 2011;103(6):520–3.

30. Tasian GE, Cooperberg MR, Potter MB, et al. PSA screening: determinants of primary-care physician practice patterns. Prostate Cancer Prostatic Dis 2012;15(2):189–94.

31. Cohn JA, Wang CE, Lakeman JC, et al. Primary care physician PSA screening practices before and after the final US Preventive Services Task Force recommendation. Urol Oncol 2014;32(1):41.e23–30.

32. Pollack CE, Noronha G, Green GE, et al. Primary care providers' response to the US Preventive Services Task Force draft recommendations on screening for prostate cancer. Arch Intern Med 2012;172(8):668–70.

33. Allen JD, Othus MK, Hart A Jr, et al. Do men make informed decisions about prostate cancer screening? Baseline results from the "take the wheel" trial. Med Decis Making 2011;31(1):108–20.

34. Hall IJ, Taylor YJ, Ross LE, et al. Discussions about prostate cancer screening between US primary care physicians and their patients. J Gen Intern Med 2011;26(10):1098–104.

35. Committee on Quality of Health Care in America, Institute of Medicine. Crossing the quality chasm: a new health system for the 21st century. Washington, DC: The National Academies Press; 2001.

36. Elwyn G, O'Connor AM, Bennett C, et al. Assessing the quality of decision support technologies using the International Patient Decision Aid Standards instrument (IPDASi). PLoS One 2009;4(3):e4705.

37. Elwyn G, O'Connor A, Stacey D, et al. Developing a quality criteria framework for patient decision aids: online international Delphi consensus process. BMJ 2006;333(7565):417.

38. Stacey D, Bennett CL, Barry MJ, et al. Decision aids for people facing health treatment or screening decisions. Cochrane Database Syst Rev 2011;(10): CD001431.

39. Volk RJ, Hawley ST, Kneuper S, et al. Trials of decision aids for prostate cancer screening: a systematic review. Am J Prev Med 2007;33(5):428–34.

40. van Vugt HA, Roobol MJ, Venderbos LD, et al. Informed decision making on PSA testing for the detection of prostate cancer: an evaluation of a leaflet with risk indicator. Eur J Cancer 2010;46(3): 669–77.

41. Frosch DL, Bhatnagar V, Tally S, et al. Internet patient decision support: a randomized controlled trial comparing alternative approaches for men considering prostate cancer screening. Arch Intern Med 2008;168(4):363–9.

42. Pignone MP, Howard K, Brenner AT, et al. Comparing 3 techniques for eliciting patient values for decision making about prostate-specific antigen screening: a randomized controlled trial. JAMA Intern Med 2013;173(5):362–8.

43. Jimbo M, Rana GK, Hawley S, et al. What is lacking in current decision aids on cancer screening? CA Cancer J Clin 2013;63(3):193–214.

44. O'Connor AM, Mulley AG Jr, Wennberg JE. Standard consultations are not enough to ensure decision quality regarding preference-sensitive options. J Natl Cancer Inst 2003;95(8):570–1.

45. Hsu C, Liss DT, Westbrook EO, et al. Incorporating patient decision aids into standard clinical practice in an integrated delivery system. Med Decis Making 2013;33(1):85–97.

46. Chan EC, McFall SL, Byrd TL, et al. A community-based intervention to promote informed decision making for prostate cancer screening among Hispanic American men changed knowledge and role preferences: a cluster RCT. Patient Educ Couns 2011;84(2):e44–51.

47. Landrey AR, Matlock DD, Andrews L, et al. Shared decision making in prostate-specific antigen testing: the effect of a mailed patient flyer prior to an annual exam. J Prim Care Community Health 2013;4(1):67–74.

Emerging PSA-Based Tests to Improve Screening

Richard J. Bryant, FRCSEd(Urol), PhD[a],
Hans Lilja, MD, PhD[a,b,c,d],*

KEYWORDS

- Prostate cancer • Detection • Screening • PSA • Kallikreins

KEY POINTS

- Using prostate-specific antigen (PSA) derivatives and additional kallikrein markers for prostate cancer diagnosis can improve the current performance characteristics of the PSA test alone.
- An improved screening test may dramatically reduce the number of men undergoing an unnecessary biopsy while maintaining the ability to detect high-risk prostate cancer.
- The use of an improved screening test may reduce both overdiagnosis and overtreatment of prostate cancer.

INTRODUCTION

Prostate cancer is the most commonly diagnosed malignancy in men in the United States. It was estimated that during 2013 in the United States, some 238,590 new prostate cancer cases would be diagnosed and 29,720 men would die from this disease.[1] Both early detection and treatment of clinically localized prostate cancer represent the most likely strategies that will enable clinicians to reduce the high rate of prostate cancer-related deaths. Prostate-specific antigen (PSA)-based testing has been widely used to aid prostate cancer detection since the late 1980s and prostate cancer-specific mortality has decreased because of PSA-based screening programs in recent years. However, there is a concern that this decline has come at the expense of overdiagnosis and overtreatment. This article provides an overview of emerging PSA-based biomarkers with the potential to improve the performance of prostate cancer screening programs.

PSA-BASED SCREENING FOR PROSTATE CANCER

The term screening describes the diagnosis of preclinical cases of a disease at an early stage to improve the outcomes for that condition. PSA-based screening for prostate cancer has to justify several important requirements to be acceptable and thereby become widely adopted by health care providers. Several recent studies have demonstrated that clear survival benefits may occur because of population-based prostate cancer screening programs using PSA.[2,3] Moreover, there is recent evidence that measuring a man's PSA level in early midlife identifies a smaller subset of men who are at risk of developing metastatic prostate cancer several decades later. For example, men with a PSA level in the highest decile at age 45 to 55 years have a tenfold or higher risk of metastatic cancer 15 to 25 years later compared with men with a PSA level below the age-median.[4] Similarly, a single PSA

[a] Nuffield Department of Surgical Sciences, John Radcliffe Hospital, University of Oxford, Headley Way, Headington, Oxford OX3 9DU, UK; [b] Department of Laboratory Medicine, Memorial Sloan-Kettering Cancer Center, 1275 York Avenue (Mailbox 213), New York, NY 10065, USA; [c] Department of Surgery (Urology), Memorial Sloan-Kettering Cancer Center, 1275 York Avenue (Mailbox 213), New York, NY 10065, USA; [d] Department of Medicine (GU-Oncology), Memorial Sloan-Kettering Cancer Center, 1275 York Avenue (Mailbox 213), New York, NY 10065, USA
* Corresponding author. Nuffield Department of Surgical Sciences, John Radcliffe Hospital, University of Oxford, Headley Way, Headington, Oxford OX3 9DU, UK.
E-mail addresses: liljah@mskcc.org; hans.lilja@nds.ox.ac.uk

Urol Clin N Am 41 (2014) 267–276
http://dx.doi.org/10.1016/j.ucl.2014.01.003

measurement at age 60 years may be very informative in predicting which men are at significant future risk of prostate cancer-specific death.[5] However, despite the clear survival benefits that arise because of PSA-based prostate cancer screening, there are several disadvantages to the widespread adoption of this practice, including the potential for overdiagnosis and subsequent overtreatment of men.[2,3,6]

Overdiagnosis and overtreatment of insignificant prostate cancers unlikely to become clinically apparent during a man's lifetime are significant problems.[7] The European Randomized Study of Screening for Prostate Cancer (ERSPC) showed that PSA-based screening can reduce prostate cancer-specific mortality by 20% within 9 years, but large numbers of men need to be screened for each life saved.[6] Further follow-up to 11 years demonstrated a greater reduction in prostate cancer-specific mortality and an improvement in the numbers needed to screen and treat to save each life.[2]

Unfortunately, PSA has several performance limitations when it is used for prostate cancer screening, including a lack of specificity. As the specificity of PSA alone is limited, a prostate biopsy is positive in only around 25% of men with a PSA between 2 and 10 ng/mL.[8] Data reported using the control arm of participants in the Prostate Cancer Prevention Trial (PCPT) clearly demonstrated that there is no absolute lower limit of PSA below which there is no risk of detecting prostate cancer at biopsy among men aged 62 to 91.[9] It is worthwhile noting, however, that there is a distinct difference between using the prostate biopsy endpoint of PCPT versus the prostate cancer metastasis or cancer death endpoints used in recent reports describing PSA-based testing.[4] A further downside of using the PSA level alone in prostate cancer screening is that no single PSA cut-off threshold has particularly good test performance characteristics.[6,10–12] Because PSA is an organ-specific, instead of a prostate cancer-specific biomarker, most men with an elevated level of PSA do not have prostate cancer. Men with a raised PSA may, therefore, be subjected to an unnecessary prostate biopsy and be exposed to the potential complications of this procedure along with considerable associated anxiety. Moreover, as explained above, some men with a low PSA result may actually have prostate cancer.[9] Many screen-detected prostate cancers may not actually require treatment, hence there is a need for a marker that can help to identify high-risk prostate cancer at an early stage, thereby enabling clinicians to undertake radical treatment enabling cure of those patients with the greatest risk of developing morbidity or mortality because of this malignancy.

Given the clear limitations of PSA-based testing for prostate cancer, there are several concerns regarding the routine use of this test within the context of a national prostate cancer screening program. Currently, around half of all men in the United States undergo regular PSA testing[13–15] and more than 1 million prostate biopsies are performed per annum in the United States alone.[16] The US Preventative Services Task Force has recently recommended against PSA-based screening for prostate cancer.[17] This announcement has caused considerable controversy in the United States and concerns have been raised regarding the methodology used to review the evidence base for screening, together with the interpretation of this evidence. One approach to improve the benefit to cost ratio of a prostate cancer screening program would be to focus more on those men with the highest risk of developing clinically significant malignancy.[5] Another strategy would be to improve methods of detection, perhaps by identifying novel diagnostic tests with a greater positive predictive value than the currently used PSA test.

PSA

Prostate cancer is an example of a urological malignancy that has benefitted from the discovery and application of a tumor marker. PSA, or human kallikrein 3 (hK3, KLK3), was discovered in 1979 and first applied to clinical use in the late 1980s and early 1990s.[12,18–28] The PSA-era has led to a greater detection of nonpalpable clinically localized disease and this has resulted in a subsequent reduction in prostate cancer-specific mortality.[29–32]

PSA is a 33-kD glycoprotein and serine protease produced under androgen-regulation[33,34] by the luminal cells of the prostate epithelium.[35–37] PSA acts to liquefy semen after ejaculation[38–42] and it is normally found in serum at low concentrations compared with the amount within the ejaculate. Several different molecular forms of PSA can be found within serum where around 70% of PSA is bound as complexed PSA (cPSA) in association with molecules such as α1-antichymotrypsin (ACT, *SERPINA3*) or macroglobulin (A2M).[41,43–48] PSA bound to ACT, but not A2M, represents the largest proportion of bound PSA that remains detectable with immunologic assays[49,50] and free inactive PSA (fPSA) is also detectable.[46] The development of antibodies specific for fPSA and cPSA has enabled accurate assays for the particular forms of PSA to be developed[46,48] so that the percentage of fPSA can be measured and used to try and improve the accuracy of prostate cancer detection.[8,43,51–56]

PSA also exists as several different isoforms. Luminal prostate epithelial cells produce proPSA, an inactive precursor of PSA that has a 7-amino-acid leader sequence. This is cleaved by the protease action of human kallikrein 2 (hK2) and other kallikreins resulting in the 237-amino-acid mature form of PSA.[57–63] Numerous truncated or clipped forms of proPSA may arise due to the incomplete removal of the 7-amino-acid leader sequence. These and other forms of PSA may be released more freely within the circulation of men with prostate cancer.[61–73] It has recently been demonstrated that the levels of [-2] proPSA are higher in prostate cancer than the benign setting and that the use of this biomarker significantly improves the rate of cancer detection compared with using total PSA (tPSA) and the free-to-total PSA ratio.[66,74–87] Intact PSA describes an intact and inactive form of proPSA that does not form a complex and which is released from prostate cancer cells.[69,73,88] In fact, it is now known that prostate cancer cells actually produce less PSA than benign epithelial cells; however, changes in the architecture of the prostate epithelium arising from malignant progression[23,26,89] result in the serum PSA level becoming elevated in many, though not all, of these men.

Because PSA is organ-specific and not prostate cancer-specific there is a considerable degree of overlap in PSA levels between patients with benign pathologies,[21,26,90–93] such as prostatitis, benign prostate hyperplasia, or urinary retention, compared with patients with prostate cancer.[28,94] A normal level of PSA was previously described as being below 4.0 ng/mL for men aged 50 to 80 years without prostate disease.[95] However, recently, it has become clear that there is no such thing as a normal PSA in terms of prostate cancer risk. Moreover, there is no PSA cut-off threshold below which the risk of detecting a prostate cancer on biopsy is zero,[9] so the choice of a PSA threshold at which a clinician might recommend a patient biopsy is controversial.[96–98] If the PSA threshold is set too high, clinically significant prostate cancers might be missed. Conversely, if it is set too low then an unacceptably high number of men without prostate cancer would be subjected to an unnecessary biopsy and, thereby, be exposed to the inherent risks and anxieties associated with this invasive procedure. The use of several PSA derivatives, such as PSA density, PSA velocity, age-adjusted PSA, free-to-total PSA ratio, and different molecular derivatives of PSA has led to various refinements in the performance of the PSA test.[53]

Despite this, the limited sensitivity and specificity of PSA means that there remains an urgent need to identify prostate cancer biomarkers with better performance characteristics than PSA alone.

ADDITIONAL HUMAN KALLIKREINS AS TUMOR MARKERS

In addition to PSA, 14 other human kallikrein-related peptidases have now been identified and structurally characterized. Human kallikrein-related peptidase 2 (hK2, KLK2) is a protease with several similarities to PSA. For example there is 80% identity in primary structure between hK2 and PSA, the expression of both the KLK2 and KLK3 genes is regulated by the signaling activity of the androgen receptor (AR) stimulated by the supply of androgens, and both PSA and hK2 display a similar and highly extensive degree of prostate-specific expression pattern. hK2 is a trypsin-like serine protease responsible for cleaving proPSA into its enzymatically active form during a cascade reaction which regulates seminal clot liquefaction. Although the concentration of hK2 in serum is about two orders of magnitude lower than that of PSA, the development of reliable assays for hK2 suggests that this kallikrein may potentially be used as a prostate cancer biomarker.[58,72,99–110] Interestingly, whereas PSA is strongly expressed in benign epithelium, hK2 becomes strongly expressed in malignant tissue, particularly in high-grade prostate cancer cases.[99,111–113] Compared with individuals without prostate cancer, men with this malignancy have higher levels of hK2 in their serum and there is reasonable correlation between the serum level of hK2 and the aggressiveness of prostate cancer present in an individual.[101,112]

Many of the kallikreins interact with each other within both normal physiologic pathways and during the development of prostate pathology. Several of the recently described kallikreins, including KLK4, KLK5, KLK6, KLK8, KLK10, KLK11, and KLK14, have been tested as potential prostate cancer biomarkers in relatively small numbers of patients.[114–120] To date, however, these additional kallikreins have not been proven clinically useful.

The kallikreins can be subject to degradation if samples undergo repeated freeze-thaw cycles, and the values of both free and intact PSA are lowered if samples are repeatedly frozen and thawed.[73,121] In general, the plasma or serum should be separated from the cellular component of blood within around 1 hour of blood draw. fPSA in serum should be assayed within the same working day, whereas plasma-based assays should be undertaken within a day or two,[105] given that there is evidence to suggest that kallikreins are more stable in plasma than in serum samples. Subsequently, the samples should be stored at $-80°C$ and repeated freeze-thaw cycles should be avoided. In general, the performance characteristics of different PSA isoforms and novel kallikreins as prostate cancer biomarkers may be optimized by the correct handling and use of clinical samples.[122]

THE USE OF COMBINATORIAL PANELS OF KALLIKREIN BIOMARKERS

In recent years, there has been interest in developing a prostate cancer screening test based on the use of assays for several kallikreins in combination. This is based on the principle that the use of a panel of biomarkers might outperform the use of PSA alone. As an example, a panel of four kallikrein markers measured in blood has been demonstrated to outperform the use of PSA alone in predicting the outcome of a prostate biopsy in several cohorts of men enrolled in randomized studies of screening.[121,123–127] Specifically, these include fPSA, single-chain intact PSA (iPSA), tPSA, and hK2. Importantly, it has become apparent that predicting biopsy outcome based on this panel of four kallikrein markers may be better than using total PSA alone in both previously screened[125–127] and hitherto unscreened[121,123,124] men. Crucially, in terms of developing a test that might be applicable to a population-based screening program for prostate cancer, the four kallikrein marker panel has the potential to dramatically reduce the number of unnecessary biopsies conducted as part of the screening program. If the four kallikrein marker panel was used in a screening program along with a man's age, regardless of whether a digital rectal examination (DRE) is incorporated, evidence suggests that the number of unnecessary biopsies can be greatly reduced without missing many high-grade cancers.[121,123,128]

Studies of the four kallikrein markers have facilitated the development of mathematical laboratory models (based on assays of the four kallikrein-markers and a man's age) and clinical models (using the four kallikreins, a man's age, and the findings at DRE). A laboratory model is potentially very useful because men within a screening program do not have to undergo a DRE, and raises the concept of the use of a finger-prick blood test, which may be performed at home or in the office, instead of a visit to a particular screening center and a clinical examination. The adoption of a simpler and less intrusive test may raise compliance with the screening program. Fortunately, assays for tPSA and fPSA are now widely available and assays for iPSA and hK2 have now been developed; therefore, all four assays could be readily and conveniently incorporated into a single test with a relatively low cost.

The performance of fewer unnecessary prostate biopsies clearly has potential benefits such as a reduction in costs, a reduced risk of biopsy-associated complications such as bleeding and sepsis, and a reduction in the anxiety experienced by men who undergo screening. An additional potential benefit to undertaking fewer biopsies within a screening program might be that fewer clinically insignificant prostate cancers are detected, thereby reducing the associated problems of over-diagnosis and overtreatment of low-grade cancers that are otherwise considered overdiagnosed using current PSA-based detection methods.[121,123] However, undertaking fewer prostate biopsies within a fixed population of screened men and thereby detecting fewer overall cancers, might be expected to result in the underdetection of clinically significant cancer cases. In fact, the available evidence from the studies performed thus far suggests that very few high-grade prostate cancers seem to be missed using the four kallikrein marker panel during an initial round of screening.[121,123] In addition, it might be reasonable to assume that any high-grade cancers potentially missed by a round of screening using the four kallikrein panel could subsequently be detected during a further round of screening. This would still be within a "window of curability," provided the screening rounds were sufficiently frequent to pick up any progressing malignancy before it had become incurable. All of the studies performed to date to evaluate the four kallikrein panel of biomarkers have been performed in European population cohorts using serum samples; however, plasma-EDTA anticoagulated samples may be more beneficial because they can be shipped to other centers for novel biomarkers to be evaluated in other laboratories. Moreover, validation studies performed using cohorts of men from the United States are needed to verify the applicability of this test in these populations. The four kallikrein marker assay is not yet readily available in the United States; however, it is likely to be introduced in the near future.

The use of different PSA isoforms and additional kallikreins as newer biomarkers within the context of a screening program has the potential to improve on the diagnostic performance of using PSA alone, resulting in fewer men needing to undergo a prostate biopsy procedure. Although the four kallikrein marker panel for example has shown particular promise in retrospective studies, many of the cohorts in the studies reported to date comprise serum, instead of plasma, samples, and many of the protocols within these screening studies included the use of sextant rather than extended core biopsies. It is now recognized that the use of extended core biopsies to detect prostate cancer is superior to sextant samples due to improved sampling of the gland.[129] Moreover, many of the studies of PSA-based screening for prostate cancer have included men in the eighth decade of life, whereas it is now recognized that the men who are likely to benefit the most from prostate cancer screening are those in earlier midlife, perhaps between the ages of 40 and 60 years. A prospective study evaluating the contemporaneous use of a panel of PSA variants and additional kallikreins, focusing on early middle-aged men with the most to gain from a well-performing screening test, would be extremely helpful in clarifying the clinical usefulness of such a panel of kallikrein biomarkers.

A novel approach to improve the clinical performance of PSA is to combine the results of three automated blood tests (tPSA, fPSA, and [-2] proPSA) using a mathematical formula termed the Prostate Health Index (phi). The phi test specifically uses the formula ([-2] proPSA/fPSA $\times$ $\sqrt{tPSA}$) to calculate and report a phi result, which can improve the rate of prostate cancer detection compared with either tPSA or f/tPSA alone.[74–77,81,83,84,87] Levels of phi have been demonstrated to differ significantly between men with and without prostate cancer in European cohorts.[84] The phi had clinical specificities of 23% and 31% at a sensitivity of 95% and 90%, compared with specificities of 10% and 8% for tPSA alone.[84] The phi has also been prospectively evaluated in a large cohort of men in the United States with PSA levels of 2 to 10 ng/mL.[74] The performance of phi was compared with tPSA, fPSA, and [-2] proPSA. At a sensitivity of 80% to 95%, the specificity of phi to detect prostate cancer was higher than for tPSA and fPSA.[74] The phi has also been shown to be a stronger predictor of prostate cancer at biopsy in men with PSA levels of 2 to 10 ng/mL in an Italian study.[75]

Use of the phi may help to reduce the number of unnecessary prostate biopsies undertaken in men with moderately elevated levels of PSA and it may provide a useful tool in the discrimination of insignificant and aggressive prostate cancer. As an example, around three-quarters of prostate cancers detected with a phi value less than 25 have been found to be clinically insignificant at prostate biopsy.[74] The phi has also been demonstrated to miss fewer prostate cancers with a Gleason score greater than 7 compared with tPSA or free-to-total

PSA,[84] whereas the risk of detecting a clinically aggressive cancer has been shown to be increased in men with higher phi readings.[74] Studies have also shown an association between phi and [-2] proPSA levels and Gleason score, suggesting that these biomarkers may be useful in the prediction of aggressive disease.[75] Whereas the level of PSA is known to correlate with prostate volume, the phi reading has been shown to correlate with tumor volume, providing further evidence that this tool may be helpful in the detection of clinically aggressive disease at prostate biopsy. By helping to reduce the number of unnecessary prostate biopsies, the use of phi not only provides a clinical benefit to men at lower levels of PSA but it can also facilitate substantial cost savings for health care systems.[130] Taken together, the available evidence suggests that phi may play an important role in the identification of prostate cancer at biopsy, especially in men more than 50 years old with a negative DRE and a tPSA in the range of 2 to 10 ng/mL. Following a prospective multicenter Food and Drug Administration (FDA) registration study, which included men with contemporary and more extensive biopsy schemes, the phi has now been approved by the FDA in the United States.

SUMMARY

Although the use of PSA has revolutionized the detection and treatment of prostate cancer, there remains considerable scope for both improvements in the use of variations of the PSA test and the development of novel biomarkers. The use of PSA derivatives and additional kallikrein markers has the potential to improve the current performance characteristics of the PSA test alone. The use of PSA as part of a multivariable approach to early prostate cancer detection, including such tools as the phi test, has recently been supported by the Melbourne Consensus Statement on Prostate Cancer Testing.[131] An improved screening test may dramatically reduce the number of men undergoing an unnecessary biopsy while maintaining the ability to detect high-risk cases of this common malignancy. Such an approach has the potential to reduce the overdiagnosis and overtreatment of prostate cancer while enabling clinicians to focus on high-risk cases of localized prostate cancer in a population of men likely to benefit from radical intervention.

REFERENCES

1. Siegel R, Naishadham D, Jemal A. Cancer statistics, 2013. CA Cancer J Clin 2013;63(1):11–30.

2. Hugosson J, Carlsson S, Aus G, et al. Mortality results from the Goteborg randomised population-based prostate-cancer screening trial. Lancet Oncol 2010;11(8):725–32.

3. Schroder FH, Hugosson J, Roobol MJ, et al. Prostate-cancer mortality at 11 years of follow-up. N Engl J Med 2012;366(11):981–90.

4. Vickers AJ, Ulmert D, Sjoberg DD, et al. Strategy for detection of prostate cancer based on relation between prostate specific antigen at age 40-55 and long term risk of metastasis: case-control study. BMJ 2013;346:f2023.

5. Vickers AJ, Lilja H. Predicting prostate cancer many years before diagnosis: how and why? World J Urol 2012;30(2):131–5.

6. Schroder FH, Hugosson J, Roobol MJ, et al. Screening and prostate-cancer mortality in a randomized European study. N Engl J Med 2009; 360(13):1320–8.

7. Welch HG, Albertsen PC. Prostate cancer diagnosis and treatment after the introduction of prostate-specific antigen screening: 1986-2005. J Natl Cancer Inst 2009;101(19):1325–9.

8. Catalona WJ, Partin AW, Slawin KM, et al. Use of the percentage of free prostate-specific antigen to enhance differentiation of prostate cancer from benign prostatic disease: a prospective multicenter clinical trial. JAMA 1998;279(19):1542–7.

9. Thompson IM, Pauler DK, Goodman PJ, et al. Prevalence of prostate cancer among men with a prostate-specific antigen level < or =4.0 ng per milliliter. N Engl J Med 2004;350(22):2239–46.

10. Lilja H, Ulmert D, Vickers AJ. Prostate-specific antigen and prostate cancer: prediction, detection and monitoring. Nat Rev Cancer 2008;8(4):268–78.

11. Thompson IM, Ankerst DP, Chi C, et al. Operating characteristics of prostate-specific antigen in men with an initial PSA level of 3.0 ng/ml or lower. JAMA 2005;294(1):66–70.

12. Ulmert D, Serio AM, O'Brien MF, et al. Long-term prediction of prostate cancer: prostate-specific antigen (PSA) velocity is predictive but does not improve the predictive accuracy of a single PSA measurement 15 years or more before cancer diagnosis in a large, representative, unscreened population. J Clin Oncol 2008;26(6):835–41.

13. Drazer MW, Huo D, Schonberg MA, et al. Population-based patterns and predictors of prostate-specific antigen screening among older men in the United States. J Clin Oncol 2011;29(13):1736–43.

14. Ross LE, Taylor YJ, Richardson LC, et al. Patterns in prostate-specific antigen test use and digital rectal examinations in the Behavioral Risk Factor Surveillance System, 2002-2006. J Natl Med Assoc 2009;101(4):316–24.

15. Sirovich BE, Schwartz LM, Woloshin S. Screening men for prostate and colorectal cancer in the United States: does practice reflect the evidence? JAMA 2003;289(11):1414–20.

16. Loeb S, Carter HB, Berndt SI, et al. Complications after prostate biopsy: data from SEER-Medicare. J Urol 2011;186(5):1830–4.

17. Summaries for patients. Screening for prostate cancer: U.S. Preventive Services Task Force recommendation statement. Ann Intern Med 2012; 157(2):1–44.

18. Ablin RJ, Soanes WA, Bronson P, et al. Precipitating antigens of the normal human prostate. J Reprod Fertil 1970;22(3):573–4.

19. Chan DW, Bruzek DJ, Oesterling JE, et al. Prostate-specific antigen as a marker for prostatic cancer: a monoclonal and a polyclonal immunoassay compared. Clin Chem 1987;33(10):1916–20.

20. Kuriyama M, Wang MC, Lee CI, et al. Use of human prostate-specific antigen in monitoring prostate cancer. Cancer Res 1981;41(10):3874–6.

21. Kuriyama M, Wang MC, Papsidero LD, et al. Quantitation of prostate-specific antigen in serum by a sensitive enzyme immunoassay. Cancer Res 1980;40(12):4658–62.

22. Oesterling JE, Chan DW, Epstein JI, et al. Prostate specific antigen in the preoperative and postoperative evaluation of localized prostatic cancer treated with radical prostatectomy. J Urol 1988; 139(4):766–72.

23. Papsidero LD, Wang MC, Valenzuela LA, et al. A prostate antigen in sera of prostatic cancer patients. Cancer Res 1980;40(7):2428–32.

24. Seamonds B, Yang N, Anderson K, et al. Evaluation of prostate-specific antigen and prostatic acid phosphatase as prostate cancer markers. Urology 1986;28(6):472–9.

25. Sensabaugh GF. Isolation and characterization of a semen-specific protein from human seminal plasma: a potential new marker for semen identification. J Forensic Sci 1978;23(1):106–15.

26. Stamey TA, Yang N, Hay AR, et al. Prostate-specific antigen as a serum marker for adenocarcinoma of the prostate. N Engl J Med 1987;317(15):909–16.

27. Wang MC, Papsidero LD, Kuriyama M, et al. Prostate antigen: a new potential marker for prostatic cancer. Prostate 1981;2(1):89–96.

28. Wang MC, Valenzuela LA, Murphy GP, et al. Purification of a human prostate specific antigen. Invest Urol 1979;17(2):159–63.

29. Polascik TJ, Oesterling JE, Partin AW. Prostate specific antigen: a decade of discovery–what we have learned and where we are going. J Urol 1999; 162(2):293–306.

30. Pound CR, Partin AW, Eisenberger MA, et al. Natural history of progression after PSA elevation following radical prostatectomy. JAMA 1999;281(17):1591–7.

31. Pound CR, Walsh PC, Epstein JI, et al. Radical prostatectomy as treatment for prostate-specific

antigen-detected stage T1c prostate cancer. World J Urol 1997;15(6):373–7.

32. Stephenson RA, Stanford JL. Population-based prostate cancer trends in the United States: patterns of change in the era of prostate-specific antigen. World J Urol 1997;15(6):331–5.

33. Henttu P, Liao SS, Vihko P. Androgens up-regulate the human prostate-specific antigen messenger ribonucleic acid (mRNA), but down-regulate the prostatic acid phosphatase mRNA in the LNCaP cell line. Endocrinology 1992;130(2):766–72.

34. Young CY, Montgomery BT, Andrews PE, et al. Hormonal regulation of prostate-specific antigen messenger RNA in human prostatic adenocarcinoma cell line LNCaP. Cancer Res 1991;51(14):3748–52.

35. Diamandis EP, Yousef GM. Human tissue kallikrein gene family: a rich source of novel disease biomarkers. Expert Rev Mol Diagn 2001;1(2):182–90.

36. Diamandis EP, Yousef GM, Luo LY, et al. The new human kallikrein gene family: implications in carcinogenesis. Trends Endocrinol Metab 2000;11(2):54–60.

37. Levesque M, Hu H, D'Costa M, et al. Prostate-specific antigen expression by various tumors. J Clin Lab Anal 1995;9(2):123–8.

38. Christensson A, Laurell CB, Lilja H. Enzymatic activity of prostate-specific antigen and its reactions with extracellular serine proteinase inhibitors. Eur J Biochem 1990;194(3):755–63.

39. Lilja H. A kallikrein-like serine protease in prostatic fluid cleaves the predominant seminal vesicle protein. J Clin Invest 1985;76(5):1899–903.

40. Lilja H, Laurell CB. Liquefaction of coagulated human semen. Scand J Clin Lab Invest 1984;44(5):447–52.

41. Lilja H, Oldbring J, Rannevik G, et al. Seminal vesicle-secreted proteins and their reactions during gelation and liquefaction of human semen. J Clin Invest 1987;80(2):281–5.

42. McGee RS, Herr JC. Human seminal vesicle-specific antigen is a substrate for prostate-specific antigen (or P-30). Biol Reprod 1988;39(2):499–510.

43. Christensson A, Bjork T, Nilsson O, et al. Serum prostate specific antigen complexed to alpha 1-antichymotrypsin as an indicator of prostate cancer. J Urol 1993;150(1):100–5.

44. Christensson A, Lilja H. Complex formation between protein C inhibitor and prostate-specific antigen in vitro and in human semen. Eur J Biochem 1994;220(1):45–53.

45. Lilja H. Prostate-specific antigen: molecular forms and the human kallikrein gene family. Br J Urol 1997;79(Suppl 1):44–8.

46. Lilja H, Christensson A, Dahlen U, et al. Prostate-specific antigen in serum occurs predominantly in complex with alpha 1-antichymotrypsin. Clin Chem 1991;37(9):1618–25.

47. McCormack RT, Rittenhouse HG, Finlay JA, et al. Molecular forms of prostate-specific antigen and the human kallikrein gene family: a new era. Urology 1995;45(5):729–44.

48. Stenman UH, Leinonen J, Alfthan H, et al. A complex between prostate-specific antigen and alpha 1-antichymotrypsin is the major form of prostate-specific antigen in serum of patients with prostatic cancer: assay of the complex improves clinical sensitivity for cancer. Cancer Res 1991;51(1):222–6.

49. Brawer MK. Prostate-specific antigen: current status. CA Cancer J Clin 1999;49(5):264–81.

50. Partin AW, Brawer MK, Bartsch G, et al. Complexed prostate specific antigen improves specificity for prostate cancer detection: results of a prospective multicenter clinical trial. J Urol 2003;170(5):1787–91.

51. Lee R, Localio AR, Armstrong K, et al. A meta-analysis of the performance characteristics of the free prostate-specific antigen test. Urology 2006;67(4):762–8.

52. Partin AW, Brawer MK, Subong EN, et al. Prospective evaluation of percent free-PSA and complexed-PSA for early detection of prostate cancer. Prostate Cancer Prostatic Dis 1998;1(4):197–203.

53. Roddam AW, Duffy MJ, Hamdy FC, et al. Use of prostate-specific antigen (PSA) isoforms for the detection of prostate cancer in men with a PSA level of 2-10 ng/ml: systematic review and meta-analysis. Eur Urol 2005;48(3):386–99 [discussion: 98–9].

54. Stephan C, Jung K, Diamandis EP, et al. Prostate-specific antigen, its molecular forms, and other kallikrein markers for detection of prostate cancer. Urology 2002;59(1):2–8.

55. Veltri RW, Miller MC. Free/total PSA ratio improves differentiation of benign and malignant disease of the prostate: critical analysis of two different test populations. Urology 1999;53(4):736–45.

56. Vessella RL, Lange PH, Partin AW, et al. Probability of prostate cancer detection based on results of a multicenter study using the AxSYM free PSA and total PSA assays. Urology 2000;55(6):909–14.

57. Kumar A, Mikolajczyk SD, Goel AS, et al. Expression of pro form of prostate-specific antigen by mammalian cells and its conversion to mature, active form by human kallikrein 2. Cancer Res 1997;57(15):3111–4.

58. Kumar A, Mikolajczyk SD, Hill TM, et al. Different proportions of various prostate-specific antigen (PSA) and human kallikrein 2 (hK2) forms are present in noninduced and androgen-induced LNCaP cells. Prostate 2000;44(3):248–54.

59. Mikolajczyk SD, Grauer LS, Millar LS, et al. A precursor form of PSA (pPSA) is a component of the free PSA in prostate cancer serum. Urology 1997;50(5):710–4.

60. Mikolajczyk SD, Marker KM, Millar LS, et al. A truncated precursor form of prostate-specific antigen is a more specific serum marker of prostate cancer. Cancer Res 2001;61(18):6958–63.

61. Mikolajczyk SD, Marks LS, Partin AW, et al. Free prostate-specific antigen in serum is becoming more complex. Urology 2002;59(6):797–802.

62. Peter J, Unverzagt C, Krogh TN, et al. Identification of precursor forms of free prostate-specific antigen in serum of prostate cancer patients by immunosorption and mass spectrometry. Cancer Res 2001;61(3):957–62.

63. Zhang WM, Leinonen J, Kalkkinen N, et al. Purification and characterization of different molecular forms of prostate-specific antigen in human seminal fluid. Clin Chem 1995;41(11):1567–73.

64. Bangma CH, Wildhagen MF, Yurdakul G, et al. The value of (-7, -5)pro-prostate-specific antigen and human kallikrein-2 as serum markers for grading prostate cancer. BJU Int 2004;93(6):720–4.

65. Lein M, Semjonow A, Graefen M, et al. A multicenter clinical trial on the use of (-5, -7) pro prostate specific antigen. J Urol 2005;174(6):2150–3.

66. Martin BJ, Finlay JA, Sterling K, et al. Early detection of prostate cancer in African-American men through use of multiple biomarkers: human kallikrein 2 (hK2), prostate-specific antigen (PSA), and free PSA (fPSA). Prostate Cancer Prostatic Dis 2004;7(2):132–7.

67. Mikolajczyk SD, Catalona WJ, Evans CL, et al. Proenzyme forms of prostate-specific antigen in serum improve the detection of prostate cancer. Clin Chem 2004;50(6):1017–25.

68. Mikolajczyk SD, Millar LS, Wang TJ, et al. A precursor form of prostate-specific antigen is more highly elevated in prostate cancer compared with benign transition zone prostate tissue. Cancer Res 2000;60(3):756–9.

69. Mikolajczyk SD, Rittenhouse HG. Tumor-associated forms of prostate specific antigen improve the discrimination of prostate cancer from benign disease. Rinsho Byori 2004;52(3):223–30.

70. Mikolajczyk SD, Song Y, Wong JR, et al. Are multiple markers the future of prostate cancer diagnostics? Clin Biochem 2004;37(7):519–28.

71. Nurmikko P, Pettersson K, Piironen T, et al. Discrimination of prostate cancer from benign disease by plasma measurement of intact, free prostate-specific antigen lacking an internal cleavage site at Lys145-Lys146. Clin Chem 2001;47(8):1415–23.

72. Sokoll LJ, Chan DW, Mikolajczyk SD, et al. Proenzyme psa for the early detection of prostate cancer in the 2.5-4.0 ng/ml total psa range: preliminary analysis. Urology 2003;61(2):274–6.

73. Steuber T, Nurmikko P, Haese A, et al. Discrimination of benign from malignant prostatic disease by selective measurements of single chain, intact free prostate specific antigen. J Urol 2002;168(5):1917–22.

74. Catalona WJ, Bartsch G, Rittenhouse HG, et al. Serum pro prostate specific antigen improves cancer detection compared to free and complexed prostate specific antigen in men with prostate specific antigen 2 to 4 ng/ml. J Urol 2003;170(6 Pt 1):2181–5.

75. Catalona WJ, Partin AW, Sanda MG, et al. A multicenter study of [-2]pro-prostate specific antigen combined with prostate specific antigen and free prostate specific antigen for prostate cancer detection in the 2.0 to 10.0 ng/ml prostate specific antigen range. J Urol 2011;185(5):1650–5.

76. de Vries SH, Raaijmakers R, Blijenberg BG, et al. Additional use of [-2] precursor prostate-specific antigen and "benign" PSA at diagnosis in screen-detected prostate cancer. Urology 2005;65(5):926–30.

77. Filella X, Gimenez N. Evaluation of [-2] proPSA and Prostate Health Index (phi) for the detection of prostate cancer: a systematic review and meta-analysis. Clin Chem Lab Med 2013;51(4):729–39.

78. Guazzoni G, Lazzeri M, Nava L, et al. Preoperative prostate-specific antigen isoform p2PSA and its derivatives, %p2PSA and prostate health index, predict pathologic outcomes in patients undergoing radical prostatectomy for prostate cancer. Eur Urol 2012;61(3):455–66.

79. Guazzoni G, Nava L, Lazzeri M, et al. Prostate-specific antigen (PSA) isoform p2PSA significantly improves the prediction of prostate cancer at initial extended prostate biopsies in patients with total PSA between 2.0 and 10 ng/ml: results of a prospective study in a clinical setting. Eur Urol 2011;60(2):214–22.

80. Houlgatte A, Vincendeau S, Desfemmes F, et al. Use of [-2] pro PSA and phi index for early detection of prostate cancer: a prospective of 452 patients. Prog Urol 2011;22(5):279–83.

81. Isharwal S, Makarov DV, Sokoll LJ, et al. ProPSA and diagnostic biopsy tissue DNA content combination improves accuracy to predict need for prostate cancer treatment among men enrolled in an active surveillance program. Urology 2011;77(3)(763):e1–6.

82. Jansen FH, van Schaik RH, Kurstjens J, et al. Prostate-specific antigen (PSA) isoform p2PSA in combination with total PSA and free PSA improves diagnostic accuracy in prostate cancer detection. Eur Urol 2010;57(6):921–7.

83. Le BV, Griffin CR, Loeb S, et al. [-2]Proenzyme prostate specific antigen is more accurate than total and free prostate specific antigen in differentiating prostate cancer from benign disease in a prospective prostate cancer screening study. J Urol 2010;183(4):1355–9.

84. Makarov DV, Isharwal S, Sokoll LJ, et al. Pro-prostate-specific antigen measurements in serum and tissue are associated with treatment necessity among men enrolled in expectant management for prostate cancer. Clin Cancer Res 2009;15(23): 7316–21.

85. Sokoll LJ, Sanda MG, Feng Z, et al. A prospective, multicenter, National Cancer Institute Early Detection Research Network study of [-2]proPSA: improving prostate cancer detection and correlating with cancer aggressiveness. Cancer Epidemiol Biomarkers Prev 2010;19(5):1193–200.

86. Sokoll LJ, Wang Y, Feng Z, et al. [-2]proenzyme prostate specific antigen for prostate cancer detection: a national cancer institute early detection research network validation study. J Urol 2008;180(2):539–43 [discussion: 43].

87. Stephan C, Kahrs AM, Cammann H, et al. A [-2] proPSA-based artificial neural network significantly improves differentiation between prostate cancer and benign prostatic diseases. Prostate 2009; 69(2):198–207.

88. Nurmikko P, Vaisanen V, Piironen T, et al. Production and characterization of novel anti-prostate-specific antigen (PSA) monoclonal antibodies that do not detect internally cleaved Lys145-Lys146 inactive PSA. Clin Chem 2000;46(10):1610–8.

89. Pinzani P, Lind K, Malentacchi F, et al. Prostate-specific antigen mRNA and protein levels in laser microdissected cells of human prostate measured by real-time reverse transcriptase-quantitative polymerase chain reaction and immuno-quantitative polymerase chain reaction. Hum Pathol 2008; 39(10):1474–82.

90. Armitage TG, Cooper EH, Newling DW, et al. The value of the measurement of serum prostate specific antigen in patients with benign prostatic hyperplasia and untreated prostate cancer. Br J Urol 1988;62(6):584–9.

91. Dalton DL. Elevated serum prostate-specific antigen due to acute bacterial prostatitis. Urology 1989;33(6):465.

92. Ercole CJ, Lange PH, Mathisen M, et al. Prostatic specific antigen and prostatic acid phosphatase in the monitoring and staging of patients with prostatic cancer. J Urol 1987;138(5):1181–4.

93. Nadler RB, Humphrey PA, Smith DS, et al. Effect of inflammation and benign prostatic hyperplasia on elevated serum prostate specific antigen levels. J Urol 1995;154(2 Pt 1):407–13.

94. Partin AW, Carter HB, Chan DW, et al. Prostate specific antigen in the staging of localized prostate cancer: influence of tumor differentiation, tumor volume and benign hyperplasia. J Urol 1990; 143(4):747–52.

95. Catalona WJ, Smith DS, Ratliff TL, et al. Measurement of prostate-specific antigen in serum as a screening test for prostate cancer. N Engl J Med 1991;324(17):1156–61.

96. Carter HB. A PSA threshold of 4.0 ng/mL for early detection of prostate cancer: the only rational approach for men 50 years old and older. Urology 2000;55(6):796–9.

97. Catalona WJ, Ramos CG, Carvalhal GF, et al. Lowering PSA cutoffs to enhance detection of curable prostate cancer. Urology 2000;55(6):791–5.

98. Catalona WJ, Southwick PC, Slawin KM, et al. Comparison of percent free PSA, PSA density, and age-specific PSA cutoffs for prostate cancer detection and staging. Urology 2000;56(2):255–60.

99. Becker C, Piironen T, Kiviniemi J, et al. Sensitive and specific immunodetection of human glandular kallikrein 2 in serum. Clin Chem 2000;46(2):198–206.

100. Darson MF, Pacelli A, Roche P, et al. Human glandular kallikrein 2 (hK2) expression in prostatic intraepithelial neoplasia and adenocarcinoma: a novel prostate cancer marker. Urology 1997; 49(6):857–62.

101. Finlay JA, Evans CL, Day JR, et al. Development of monoclonal antibodies specific for human glandular kallikrein (hK2): development of a dual antibody immunoassay for hK2 with negligible prostate-specific antigen cross-reactivity. Urology 1998;51(5):804–9.

102. Klee GG, Goodmanson MK, Jacobsen SJ, et al. Highly sensitive automated chemiluminometric assay for measuring free human glandular kallikrein-2. Clin Chem 1999;45(6 Pt 1):800–6.

103. Lovgren J, Valtonen-Andre C, Marsal K, et al. Measurement of prostate-specific antigen and human glandular kallikrein 2 in different body fluids. J Androl 1999;20(3):348–55.

104. Martin BJ, Cheli CD, Sterling K, et al. Prostate specific antigen isoforms and human glandular kallikrein 2–which offers the best screening performance in a predominantly black population? J Urol 2006;175(1):104–7.

105. Nam RK, Diamandis EP, Toi A, et al. Serum human glandular kallikrein-2 protease levels predict the presence of prostate cancer among men with elevated prostate-specific antigen. J Clin Oncol 2000;18(5):1036–42.

106. Piironen T, Pettersson K, Suonpaa M, et al. In vitro stability of free prostate-specific antigen (PSA) and prostate-specific antigen (PSA) complexed to alpha 1-antichymotrypsin in blood samples. Urology 1996;48(6A Suppl):81–7.

107. Rittenhouse HG, Finlay JA, Mikolajczyk SD, et al. Human Kallikrein 2 (hK2) and prostate-specific antigen (PSA): two closely related, but distinct, kallikreins in the prostate. Crit Rev Clin Lab Sci 1998; 35(4):275–368.

108. Stephan C, Jung K, Lein M, et al. Molecular forms of prostate-specific antigen and human kallikrein

2 as promising tools for early diagnosis of prostate cancer. Cancer Epidemiol Biomarkers Prev 2000; 9(11):1133–47.

109. Young CY, Andrews PE, Montgomery BT, et al. Tissue-specific and hormonal regulation of human prostate-specific glandular kallikrein. Biochemistry 1992;31(3):818–24.

110. Yousef GM, Kyriakopoulou LG, Scorilas A, et al. Quantitative expression of the human kallikrein gene 9 (KLK9) in ovarian cancer: a new independent and favorable prognostic marker. Cancer Res 2001;61(21):7811–8.

111. Darson MF, Pacelli A, Roche P, et al. Human glandular kallikrein 2 expression in prostate adenocarcinoma and lymph node metastases. Urology 1999;53(5):939–44.

112. Kwiatkowski MK, Recker F, Piironen T, et al. In prostatism patients the ratio of human glandular kallikrein to free PSA improves the discrimination between prostate cancer and benign hyperplasia within the diagnostic "gray zone" of total PSA 4 to 10 ng/mL. Urology 1998;52(3):360–5.

113. Tremblay RR, Deperthes D, Tetu B, et al. Immunohistochemical study suggesting a complementary role of kallikreins hK2 and hK3 (prostate-specific antigen) in the functional analysis of human prostate tumors. Am J Pathol 1997;150(2):455–9.

114. Nakamura T, Mitsui S, Okui A, et al. Molecular cloning and expression of a variant form of hippostasin/KLK11 in prostate. Prostate 2003;54(4):299–305.

115. Nakamura T, Stephan C, Scorilas A, et al. Quantitative analysis of hippostasin/KLK11 gene expression in cancerous and noncancerous prostatic tissues. Urology 2003;61(5):1042–6.

116. Obiezu CV, Soosaipillai A, Jung K, et al. Detection of human kallikrein 4 in healthy and cancerous prostatic tissues by immunofluorometry and immunohistochemistry. Clin Chem 2002;48(8):1232–40.

117. Parekh DJ, Ankerst DP, Baillargeon J, et al. Assessment of 54 biomarkers for biopsy-detectable prostate cancer. Cancer Epidemiol Biomarkers Prev 2007;16(10):1966–72.

118. Sardana G, Marshall J, Diamandis EP. Discovery of candidate tumor markers for prostate cancer via proteomic analysis of cell culture-conditioned medium. Clin Chem 2007;53(3):429–37.

119. Xi Z, Klokk TI, Korkmaz K, et al. Kallikrein 4 is a predominantly nuclear protein and is overexpressed in prostate cancer. Cancer Res 2004;64(7):2365–70.

120. Yousef GM, Stephan C, Scorilas A, et al. Differential expression of the human kallikrein gene 14 (KLK14) in normal and cancerous prostatic tissues. Prostate 2003;56(4):287–92.

121. Vickers AJ, Cronin AM, Aus G, et al. A panel of kallikrein markers can reduce unnecessary biopsy for prostate cancer: data from the European Randomized Study of Prostate Cancer Screening in Goteborg, Sweden. BMC Med 2008;6:19.

122. Ulmert D, Becker C, Nilsson JA, et al. Reproducibility and accuracy of measurements of free and total prostate-specific antigen in serum vs plasma after long-term storage at -20 degrees C. Clin Chem 2006;52(2):235–9.

123. Benchikh A, Savage C, Cronin A, et al. A panel of kallikrein markers can predict outcome of prostate biopsy following clinical work-up: an independent validation study from the European Randomized Study of Prostate Cancer screening, France. BMC Cancer 2010;10:635.

124. Gupta A, Roobol MJ, Savage CJ, et al. A four-kallikrein panel for the prediction of repeat prostate biopsy: data from the European Randomized Study of Prostate Cancer screening in Rotterdam, Netherlands. Br J Cancer 2010;103(5):708–14.

125. Vickers A, Cronin A, Roobol M, et al. Reducing unnecessary biopsy during prostate cancer screening using a four-kallikrein panel: an independent replication. J Clin Oncol 2010;28(15):2493–8.

126. Vickers AJ, Cronin AM, Aus G, et al. Impact of recent screening on predicting the outcome of prostate cancer biopsy in men with elevated prostate-specific antigen: data from the European Randomized Study of Prostate Cancer Screening in Gothenburg, Sweden. Cancer 2010;116(11):2612–20.

127. Vickers AJ, Cronin AM, Roobol MJ, et al. A four-kallikrein panel predicts prostate cancer in men with recent screening: data from the European Randomized Study of Screening for Prostate Cancer, Rotterdam. Clin Cancer Res 2010;16(12):3232–9.

128. Vickers AJ, Gupta A, Savage CJ, et al. A panel of kallikrein marker predicts prostate cancer in a large, population-based cohort followed for 15 years without screening. Cancer Epidemiol Biomarkers Prev 2011;20(2):255–61.

129. European Association of Urology. Prostate cancer. Full guidelines. 2012 [cited 7th May 2013]. Available at: http://www.uroweb.org/guidelines/online-guidelines/. Accessed May 7, 2013.

130. Nichol MB, Wu J, An JJ, et al. Budget impact analysis of a new prostate cancer risk index for prostate cancer detection. Prostate Cancer Prostatic Dis 2011;14(3):253–61.

131. Murphy D. The Melbourne Consensus Statement on Prostate Cancer Testing. 2013 [cited 24th November 2013]. Available at: http://www.bjuinternational.com/bjui-blog/the-melbourne-consensus-statement-on-prostate-cancer-testing/. Accessed November 24, 2013.

The Epidemiology and Clinical Implications of Genetic Variation in Prostate Cancer

Brian T. Helfand, MD, PhD[a],*, William J. Catalona, MD[b]

KEYWORDS

- Prostate cancer • Genetic variants • Susceptibility • Tumor aggressiveness

KEY POINTS

- There is a strong genetic predisposition to prostate cancer.
- Studies have identified rare, highly penetrant genetic variants that significantly increase the risk of prostate cancer and the aggressive forms of the disease.
- Genome-wide association studies have identified common widely validated genetic variations within the population that increase the risk of prostate cancer in a cumulative fashion.
- Genetic mutations within tumors have also been found that contribute to disease risk and aggressiveness; some have been incorporated into commercial assays.
- The mechanisms by which genetic variations influence the risk and progression of prostate cancer and their clinical application are under investigation; however, these variants hold potential to improve and personalize current screening and treatment algorithms.

INTRODUCTION

Prostate cancer (PC) is the second most common visceral malignancy in men worldwide, with approximately 900,000 new cases being diagnosed annually.[1] However, there is substantial variation in disease incidence based on geographic region. This situation is partly due to the influence and variability in the implementation of routine testing for PC with serum prostate-specific antigen (PSA) measurement and digital rectal examination. As such, geographic regions with the highest rates of testing, such as the United States and Western and Northern Europe, have the highest reported rates of PC, whereas regions with low rates of testing, such as some Asian and African countries, have the lowest incidence rates.[2] In addition, in countries with high PC incidence rates, there is a significant discrepancy between PC incidence and mortality. For example, there are almost 240,000 new PC diagnoses annually in the United States, but fewer than 15% of these men ultimately die of PC.[3] This low mortality-to-incidence ratio is largely attributed to the widespread implementation of PSA testing and effective treatment of early-stage disease throughout the United States.[4–7]

Since its introduction as an aid to the early detection of PC in the 1990s, PSA testing has influenced the diagnosis and treatment of PC.[7] Routine PSA testing has been associated with a stage migration toward increased diagnoses of organ-confined, low-grade PC.[4–7] The result has been a significant decrease in both the percentage and absolute number of men presenting with metastatic disease as well as a 45% reduction in the age-adjusted PC-specific mortality rate.[8] Despite these improvements, PSA testing has negatively

Disclosures: B.T. Helfand: None; W.J. Catalona: Beckman Coulter, Inc, deCODE Genetics, Inc, Ohmx, Inc, Nanosphere, Inc.
[a] Department of Surgery, NorthShore University HealthSystem, University of Chicago Pritzker School of Medicine, 2650 Ridge Avenue, Evanston, IL 60201, USA; [b] Department of Urology, Feinberg School of Medicine, Northwestern University, 303 East Superior Avenue, Terry Building 16, Chicago, IL 60611, USA
* Corresponding author.
E-mail address: bhelfand@northshore.org

Urol Clin N Am 41 (2014) 277–297
http://dx.doi.org/10.1016/j.ucl.2014.01.001
0094-0143/14/$ – see front matter © 2014 Elsevier Inc. All rights reserved.

affected some men. It is likely that some have been subject to risks secondary to potentially unnecessary biopsies and the overtreatment of a non–life-threatening PC that may not have been diagnosed without PSA testing. Furthermore, unnecessary treatment is costly and may be associated with side effects.[9–11] Thus, there is an urgent need for new biomarkers to distinguish aggressive from indolent PC and to improve current early detection strategies and clinical treatment decisions.

The strongest risk factor for PC, other than advanced age and race (eg, African American ancestry), is family history of the disease.[12–14] In fact, it has been shown that PC is one of the most heritable of cancers, as studies of twins have shown that up to 42% of the risk can be explained by genetic factors.[15] Epidemiologic data provide further support for a hereditary component. For example, data derived from a Swedish population-based study suggested that 11.6% of PC cases can be accounted for by familial factors alone.[16] In addition, a meta-analysis investigating familial clustering suggested that risk was greater for men with affected brothers (relative risk [RR] = 3.4) than for men with affected fathers (RR = 2.2). Second-degree relatives conferred a lower risk (RR = 1.7) than fathers or brothers, and having 2 or more first-degree relatives conferred the highest risk (RR = 5.1).[17] The risk also appears to be greater among probands with first-degree relatives who are diagnosed with PC at younger ages.[18]

Until recently, the study of cancer genetics has focused on identifying a few genes with high penetrance.[14,19] Despite strong evidence for the existence of PC susceptibility genes, family-based linkage studies have largely failed to reproducibly identify mutations within genes that can explain most PC cases. This is believed to be due to the high incidence of nonfamilial PC and the lack of statistical power in familial (segregation) studies. However, over the past several decades, PC genetics has been revolutionized by increasing genetic technologies at significantly decreasing costs. Specifically, the field witnessed a progression from these early linkage studies involving families of PC patients using microsatellite markers, to loss-of-heterozygosity studies using a more targeted approach with candidate genes (eg, BRCA and retinoblastoma genes), to genome-wide association studies (GWAS) of genetic variants (called single-nucleotide polymorphisms [SNPs]), to expression profiling studies to copy number variation studies, to whole exome sequencing, and now to entire genome-sequencing studies. These advances have allowed for the identification of genetic variants in both germline and tumor DNA that increase a man's risk for PC and aggressive disease (eg, Refs.[20–22]). This review discusses the potential use of genetic markers as a way to identify groups of men at high risk of developing PC, improve screening practices, discriminate aggressive from indolent disease, and, potentially, personalize therapeutic strategies.

USEFULNESS OF RARE GENOMIC VARIATION IN SCREENING FOR AND TREATMENT OF PROSTATE CANCER

As previously mentioned, many prior genetic studies have failed to identify a highly prevalent and penetrant gene or mutation associated with PC susceptibility. Linkage studies have identified PC-risk loci on several chromosomes, with the strongest linkage being to chromosome 1. Notable candidate genes include HPC1 on chromosome 1q23-35, PCAP on chromosome 1q42-43, and CAPB on chromosome 1p36.[23] In addition, data from the International Consortium for Prostate Cancer Genetics (ICPCG) has identified 12 additional regions associated with PC risk, including 1q23, 5q11, 5q35, 6q21, 8q12, 11q13, and 20p11-q11.[24]

Many studies have revealed an association between rare mutations in the breast cancer predisposition genes (BRCA1 and BRCA2) and PC risk.[25–27] BRCA1 and BRCA2 are tumor-suppressor genes, located on chromosomes 17q21 and 13q12, respectively, that are inherited in an autosomal dominant fashion. In healthy individuals, the BRCA1 and BRCA2 genes function within the DNA repair pathway, and help regulate transcription and chromatin remodeling. However, in patients with germline mutations in one of the BRCA genes, acquired inactivated or mutation of the remaining wild-type allele is associated with tumorigenesis. This loss of function is associated with loss of DNA repair mechanisms (eg, double-strand breaks by homologous recombination) and genomic instability, which often results in tumors within breast, ovarian, pancreatic, and prostate tissue.[28–31]

One of the major challenges to studying the role of BRCA mutations in PC susceptibility is the relatively low incidence of germline mutations in those genes.[32–35] Although present in less than 0.3% of sporadic PC cases, germline mutations within the BRCA genes have been associated with a significantly increased risk of PC (for BRCA1 it is increased up to 3.5-fold, and for BRCA2 it is increased up to 8.6-fold in men ≤65 years).[33] In addition, it has been estimated that the lifetime risk of developing PC in BRCA1 or BRCA2 mutation carriers is 20% and approximately 10%, respectively.[25] These risks may be more exaggerated in certain cohorts of men, including the Ashkenazi Jewish population, in which the incidence of BRCA mutations has been estimated to be approximately 2%.[36–39]

While the evidence linking BRCA mutations to the PC risk is established there is continued debate as to the association between these mutations and aggressive PC as well as adverse clinical outcomes. However, several case-case studies have suggested an association between BRCA2 carriers and more poorly differentiated and larger tumors in comparison with noncarriers.[40,41] In addition, many recent studies have suggested a relationship between BRCA2 mutation status and less favorable overall and PC-specific survival that is independent of prognostic factors such as tumor stage, Gleason score, and PSA level.[40,42–44] Because of the association with aggressive tumors, BRCA mutation carriers identified through genotyping patients with a family history suggestive of a BRCA mutation (early-onset breast and ovarian cancer) should be screened with PSA and digital rectal examination. BRCA mutation carriers diagnosed with apparent low-risk disease may not be good candidates for active surveillance protocols, and should probably undergo radical treatment (eg, surgery or radiation).

Knowledge of a man's BRCA mutation status also may help guide therapy in men with advanced PC. For example, in a cohort of women with ovarian cancer associated with BRCA2 mutations, platinum-based chemotherapy was associated with improved outcomes.[45] For men, there is evidence that BRCA-associated PC responds to poly-ADP ribose polymerase (PARP) inhibition, suggesting that carrier status may affect treatment selection.[46,47] However, this might not be the case for all treatment options. Gallagher and colleagues[48] suggested that BRCA status might not affect outcomes in BRCA mutation carriers with advanced PC who were treated with standard chemotherapy regimens using docetaxel and glucocorticoids, when compared with a cohort of noncarriers with a comparable disease status.

Taken together, it seems that although mutations within the BRCA genes are highly penetrant and may even predispose to aggressive disease, their clinical usefulness in population-wide screening may be limited by their low incidence. Knowledge of an individual's BRCA status may help guide treatment algorithms; however, future and ongoing trials, including the IMPACT Trial (Identification of Men with a genetic Predisposition to ProstAte Cancer: Targeted screening in men at higher genetic risk and controls) will help answer how to improve both screening and treatments among men harboring BRCA mutations.

The BRCA genes are not the only DNA-repair genes associated with PC. Associations between other DNA-repair genes, including PALB2, BRIP1, CHEK22, and NBS1 genes and PC have also been recognized. In addition, while initially recognized that mutations within DNA mismatch repair genes, including MLH1, MSH2, MSH6, and PMS2, are associated with a 35% to 80% increased lifetime risk of developing colorectal cancer, it is now accepted that they also confer a significantly greater risk of other cancers, including gastric, ovarian, pancreatic, brain, and sebaceous tumors.[49,50] Most recently it was shown that these mutations also increase the risk of PC.[51,52] Da Silva and colleagues[53] analyzed a relatively small population of men and reported that more than 20% of carriers of these mutated genes developed PC. By contrast, other studies have estimated that the risk associated with these mutations is much lower, ranging between 2% and 3%.[54,55] Lynch syndrome, which involves mutated mismatch repair genes, has also been implicated in PC. A familial-based study of PC estimated that the cumulative lifetime risk of prostate cancer in individuals with Lynch syndrome is more than 2-fold higher than in the general population and is slightly higher in carriers diagnosed with early-onset PC (ie, <60 years).[51] Prospective follow-up in men with Lynch syndrome will help shed light on the natural history of PC in men with mutations within mismatch repair genes and also help to guide therapies in men with Lynch syndrome.

Mutations and variations within BRCA and many of the DNA mismatch repair gene family members are not only are associated with a greater risk of developing familial PC but also have implications in the prognosis and potential management of the disease. Genotyping for these mutations within families can be performed to help aid identification of high-risk populations. In addition, given their potential associations with aggressive and early-onset disease, carriers of these mutations may be less favorable candidates for active surveillance strategies. Future studies are needed to design personalized management of these patients.

USEFULNESS OF COMMON GENOMIC VARIATION AND SCREENING FOR PROSTATE CANCER

It has been estimated that 99.9% of the human DNA sequence is identical between any 2 individuals. However, given the vast size of the human genome (3.2 billion base pairs), even this small difference results in millions of potential genetic variations. These common variations are called SNPs and are classically defined as having a variant allele (referred to as minor allele) frequency of greater than 5%.[56] Advances in high-throughput genotyping, together with the completion of the HapMap and Human Genome Projects, have enabled the performance of GWAS and, even more recently, detailed whole-exome and whole-genome sequencing studies. These genetic studies have generally been designed as case-control studies involving relatively large cohorts of patients that evaluate associations between the frequencies of SNPs and disease status. The SNPs identified in GWAS are believed to be surrogates for the true causative locus within a linkage disequilibrium block that is biologically responsible for the association.[57]

Although many early linkage, admixture, and cytogenetic studies suggested an association between PC risk and the 8q24 region,[58–60] it was not until 2006 that a PC GWAS confirmed the association.[61] These results were validated in many different large cohorts of men and thus represent a common, reproducible variant associated with increased risk of sporadic PC, and later with familial PC as well. Rapid advances in genetics research have allowed fine-mapping studies of 8q24 that have now identified more than 8 variants located within at least 5 distinct PC susceptibility regions.[62–64] These PC-risk SNPs lie in a so-called gene desert (ie, a region of the genome that is devoid of genes), with the closest annotated gene being *MYC*, located approximately 200 to 700 kilobases away. *MYC* is considered an important oncogene in PC because the locus is often amplified in tumors, and functional experiments have shown that human *MYC* expression in the mouse prostate can lead to invasive adenocarcinoma.[65] However, it should be noted that SNPs in the *MYC* gene locus itself are not in linkage with the genetic variants associated with PC risk.[61,66] Results of several studies have suggested that the PC-risk SNPs contain functional transcriptional enhancers that physically interact with the *MYC* locus and influence *MYC* regulation.[67–69] Risk loci at 8q24 may also alter binding to the transcription factors *TCF4*, *FOXA1*, or *YY1*, which could also influence gene expression and cell behavior of PC tumor.[67,70,71]

GWAS of PC have rapidly progressed after the identification of the 8q24 locus (**Table 1**).[22,72,73] In fact, there are now almost 80 different genetic variants associated with increased PC risk identified by GWAS on 20 different chromosomes. In general, the relative increased risk of developing PC based on any individual SNP is small, ranging from 1.02- to 1.5-fold.[74] However, this risk appears to be cumulative and increases with the number of risk alleles that an individual carries.[75–78] Together with family history, it has been estimated that these SNPs can explain approximately 30% of the familial risk of PC in populations of men of European ancestry.[72]

Recent technological advances in sequencing techniques have allowed researchers to perform more detailed genetic analyses. Whole-genome and exome sequencing studies have recently revealed other relatively rare, highly penetrant genetic variants (minor allele frequency in the population ≤1%) associated with PC risk, which also have been validated in independent populations. For example, coding variants in the homeobox B13 (HOXB13) gene were recently identified through targeted exonic sequencing of genes in a region of PC linkage at chromosome 17q21-22.[24,79–81] In 4 families of European-American ancestry, a rare mutation associated with an amino acid substitution of glutamic acid for glycine was detected in *HOXB13* (G84E, rs138213197).[81] This mutation was then genotyped in a large number of additional samples, and was found in 72 of 5083 PC cases (carrier frequency = 1.4%), but in only 1 of 1401 controls (carrier frequency = 0.07%). The G84E mutation frequency was increased to 2.2% when analyses were restricted to men with early-onset disease (≤55 years) or a family history of PC.[81] Other studies have confirmed this finding in men of European ancestry, and different *HOXB13* mutations have been detected in PC cases of African American and Asian ancestry.[63,82–86] In addition, another contemporary sequencing study has documented an association between a rare, relatively highly penetrant genetic variant on chromosome 8q24 (rs188140481, A allele) that significantly increases an individual's risk of PC by almost 3-fold (odds ratio [OR] = 2.90).[63]

Given the controversy over the benefits of routine PSA testing,[8] as germline SNPs are validated markers associated with increased PC risk that do not fluctuate over time or with other concomitant disease processes, there is interest in their use as biomarkers to improve PC screening strategies. Several studies have evaluated panels of SNPs in this regard. A study involving more than 3500 PC cases and controls evaluated a panel of 5 SNPs associated with the risk of developing PC. Carriers of all 5 risk alleles who had a family history of PC had an approximately 9.5-fold increased risk for developing the disease compared with men without a family history carrying no risk alleles.[78] However, it should be noted

Table 1
List of genetic variants associated with significantly increased risk of prostate cancer

Locus	SNP	Reference Allele	Risk Allele	Per Allele OR	(95% CI)	Nearby Genes
1q21	rs1218582	A	G	1.06	(1.03–1.09)	KCNN3
1q32	rs4245739	A	C	0.91	(0.88–0.95)	MDM4, PIK3C2B
2p11	rs10187424	A	G	0.92	(0.89–0.94)	GGCX/VAMP8
2p15	rs721048	G	A	1.15	(1.10–1.21)	EHBP1
2p21	rs1465618	G	A	1.08	(1.03–1.12)	THADA
2p24	rs13385191	A	G	1.15	(1.10–1.21)	C2orf43
2p25	rs11902236	G	A	1.07	(1.03–1.10)	TAF1B:GRHL1
2q31	rs12621278	A	G	0.75	(0.70–0.80)	ITGA6
2q37	rs2292884	A	G	1.14	(1.09–1.19)	MLPH
2q37	rs3771570	G	A	1.12	(1.08–1.17)	FARP2
3p11	rs2055109	T	C	1.2	(1.13–1.29)	Unknown
3p12	rs2660753	C	T	1.18	(1.06–1.31)	Unknown
3q13	rs7611694	A	C	0.91	(0.88–0.93)	SIDT1
3q21	rs10934853	C	A	1.12	(1.08–1.16)	EEFSEC
3q23	rs6763931	C	T	1.04	(1.01–1.07)	ZBTB38
3q26	rs10936632	A	C	0.9	(0.88–0.93)	CLDN11/SKIL
4q13	rs1894292	G	A	0.91	(0.89–0.94)	AFM, RASSF6
4q22	rs17021918	C	T	0.9	(0.87–0.93)	PDLIM5
4q22	rs12500426	C	A	1.08	(1.05–1.12)	PDLIM5
4q24	rs7679673	C	A	0.91	(0.88–0.94)	TET2
5p12	rs2121875	T	G	1.05	(1.02–1.08)	FGF10
5p15	rs2736098	G	A	0.87	(0.84–0.90)	TERT
5p15	rs12653946	C	T	1.26	(1.20–1.33)	IRX4
5p15CL	rs401681	G	A	1.07	(0.86–1.33)	CLPTM1
5q35	rs6869841	G	A	1.07	(1.04–1.11)	FAM44B (BOD1)
6p21	rs130067	T	G	1.05	(1.02–1.09)	CCHCR1
6p21	rs1983891	C	T	1.15	(1.09–1.21)	FOXP4
6p21	rs3096702	G	A	1.07	(1.04–1.10)	NOTCH4
6p21	rs2273669	A	G	1.07	(1.03–1.11)	ARMC2, SESN1
6q22	rs339331	C	T	1.22	(1.15–1.28)	RFX6
6q25	rs9364554	C	T	1.17	(1.08–1.26)	SLC22A3
6q25	rs1933488	A	G	0.89	(0.87–0.92)	RSG17
7p15	rs10486567	A	G	0.74	(0.66–0.83)	JAZF1
7p21	rs12155172	G	A	1.11	(1.07–1.15)	SP8
7q21	rs6465657	T	C	1.12	(1.05–1.20)	LMTK2
8p21	rs2928679	C	T	1.05	(1.01–1.09)	SLC25A37
8p21	rs1512268	G	A	1.18	(1.14–1.22)	NKX3.1
8p21	rs11135910	G	A	1.11	(1.07–1.16)	EBF2
8q24	rs188140481	G	A	2.90	(2.44–3.44)	Unknown
8q24	rs1447295	C	A	1.62	(1.20–1.93)	Unknown
8q24	rs6983267	T	G	1.26	(1.13–1.41)	Unknown
8q24	rs16901979	C	A	1.79	(1.36–2.34)	Unknown
8q24	rs10086908	T	C	0.87	(0.81–0.94)	Unknown
8q24	rs16902094	G	A	1.21	(1.15–1.26)	Unknown

(continued on next page)

Table 1
(continued)

Locus	SNP	Reference Allele	Risk Allele	Per Allele OR	(95% CI)	Nearby Genes
8q24	rs445114	C	T	1.22	(1.12–1.32)	Unknown
8q24	rs12543663	A	C	1.08	(1.00–1.16)	Unknown
8q24	rs620861	C	T	0.9	(0.84–0.96)	Unknown
9q31	rs817826	T	C	1.41	(1.29–1.54)	RAD23B-KLF4
9q33	rs1571801	C	A	1.27	(1.10–1.48)	DAB21P
10q11	rs10993994	C	T	1.25	(1.17–1.34)	MSMB
10q24	rs3850699	A	G	0.91	(0.89–0.94)	TRIM8
10q26	rs4962416	T	C	1.2	(1.07–1.34)	CTBP2
10q26	rs2252004	T	G	1.16	(1.10–1.22)	Unknown
11p15	rs7127900	G	A	1.22	(1.17–1.27)	Unknown
11q12	rs1938781	T	C	1.16	(1.11–1.21)	FAM111A
11q13	rs11228565	G	A	1.23	(1.16–1.31)	TPCN2-MYEOV
11q13	rs10896450	A	G	1.16	(1.06–1.27)	TPCN2-MYEOV
11q13	rs12418451	G	A	1.15	(1.06–1.24)	Unknown
11q13	rs7931342	G	T	0.84	(0.79–0.90)	Unknown
11q22	rs11568818	A	G	0.91	(0.88–0.94)	MMP7
12q13	rs10875943	T	C	1.07	(1.04–1.10)	TUBA1C/PRPH
12q13	rs902774	G	A	1.17	(1.11–1.24)	KRT8
12q24	rs1270884	G	A	1.07	(1.04–1.10)	TBX5
13q22	rs9600079	G	T	1.18	(1.12–1.24)	Unknown
14q22	rs8008270	G	A	0.89	(0.86–0.93)	FERMT2
14q24	rs7141529	A	G	1.09	(1.06–1.12)	RAD51L1
17p13	rs684232	A	G	1.1	(1.07–1.14)	VPS53, FAM57A
17q12	rs4430796	G	A	1.22	(1.15–1.30)	HNF1B
17q12	rs11649743	A	G	1.28	(1.07–1.52)	HNF1B
17q21	rs138213197	G	A	20.1	(3.5–803.3)	HOXB13
17q21	rs7210100	A	G	1.51	(1.35–1.69)	ZNF652
17q21	rs11650494	G	A	1.15	(1.09–1.22)	SPOP, HOXB13
17q24	rs1859962	T	G	1.2	(1.14–1.27)	Unknown
18q23	rs7241993	G	A	0.92	(0.89–0.95)	SALL3
19q13	rs2735839	G	A	0.83	(0.75–0.91)	KLK2/KLK3
19q13	rs8102476	T	C	1.12	(1.08–1.15)	Unknown
19q13	rs11672691	G	A	1.12	(1.03–1.21)	Unknown
19q13	rs103294	T	C	1.28	(1.21–1.36)	LILRA3
20q13	rs2427345	G	A	0.94	(0.91–0.97)	GATAS, CABLES2
20q13	rs6062509	A	C	0.89	(0.66–0.92)	ZGPAT
22q13	rs9623117	A	C	1.18	(1.11–1.26)	TNRC6B
22q13	rs5759167	G	T	0.86	(0.83–0.88)	BIL/TTLL1
Xp11	rs5945572	T	C	1.23	(1.16–1.30)	NUDT11
Xp22	rs2405942	A	G	0.88	(0.83–0.92)	SHROOM2
Xq12	rs5919432	A	G	0.94	(0.89–0.98)	AR

Abbreviations: CI, confidence interval; OR, odds ratio; SNP, single-nucleotide polymorphism.
Data from Refs.[61–63,66,72,103,137,172,216–221]

that those carrying either no or all risk SNPs represented only a small subset of the cohort studied. Overall, the 5-SNP-panel genotype was not able to contribute significantly to PC-risk prediction after adjusting for established risk factors such as age or family history.[78] In a later study that examined the first 14 PC-risk–associated SNPs identified in various GWAS studies, 55-year-old men with a family history of PC who also were carriers of all 14 risk alleles were found to have a 52% risk of being diagnosed with PC over a 20-year period. In comparison, without the knowledge of the SNP genotype and family history, these men would have been predicted to have an average population absolute risk of 13%.[87] Similarly, many other studies have demonstrated a cumulative effect of PC risk with panels of varying numbers of SNPs in different cohorts of men.[75–77,88–91] The cumulative level of PC risk as predicted by associated risk SNPs is comparable with current population risk screening methods for various other types of cancer, such as screening for lung cancer based on smoking status, or screening for breast cancer based on mammography.[92,93]

Other studies have recently evaluated larger and different panels of SNPs that have been validated for PC diagnosis on biopsy. It has been shown that when combined with clinical characteristics such as family history or PSA, the PC-risk SNPs can significantly improve the prediction of biopsy results. For example, a recent GWAS demonstrated that a panel of 23 PC-risk SNPs can be used in combination with PSA to significantly improve the prediction of prostate biopsy outcomes.[94] Similarly, using a Swedish cohort of men who underwent a prostate biopsy during the period 2005 to 2007, it was shown that a genetic prediction model that included PC-risk SNPs and existing clinical variables (age, PSA, free-to-total PSA, and family history) performed significantly better than the clinical model only.[95] The genetic model group required significantly fewer biopsies than the group not using the genetic model (22.7%), at a cost of missing a PC diagnosis in 3% of patients with aggressive disease characteristics.[95] These results suggest the genetic markers can be used to improve risk prediction, and ultimately may help reduce the number of unnecessary biopsies performed.

The potential benefit of applying all known PC SNPs to routine clinical practice has yet to be evaluated. To date, no study has evaluated the usefulness of a panel of the nearly 80 different PC-risk SNPs or some of the rarer genetic variants in this regard. Although it is possible that a panel of SNPs may benefit a relatively small population of men who are carriers of a majority of SNPs, it is likely that more would benefit in the future as new risk SNPs continue to be identified. Thus, as knowledge of the SNPs increases, genotyping could result in more efficient screening protocols.

Marked genetic variation exists between men of different races, and most PC-risk SNPs were identified in populations of European ancestry. Although men of African heritage are at a far higher risk of developing PC and dying of PC, fewer PC GWAS have been performed in African Americans.[96–100] However, several studies have been performed in both African and African American cohorts.[99,101–109] In general, these studies suggest that while some of the same European PC-risk SNPs are associated with increased susceptibility in black men, many do not. Future genetic studies in African Americans and other ethnically diverse populations are critical to the understanding of PC, and also will help identify risk factors that can be used to improve outcomes in all populations.

USEFULNESS OF COMMON GENOMIC VARIATION TO IMPROVE CURRENT SERUM PSA SCREENING

The most commonly used screening test for PC is measurement of the serum concentration of PSA. However, there is no single threshold value for PSA that can reliably distinguish patients with PC from those without. Thus, many men without PC, but with high PSA levels, are subjected to the morbidities associated with diagnostic biopsies. As such, there has been a large research effort into improving the performance of PSA testing itself, including measuring PSA isoforms.[110] Recently it has been shown that genetic factors can also be used to improve the performance characteristics of PSA testing.[94,111]

It has previously been estimated that 40% to 45% of the interindividual variability in measured serum PSA concentrations can be explained by genetic factors.[112,113] Recent studies have shown that SNPs in or near the gene that encodes PSA (eg, kallikrein-related peptidase 3 [KLK3]) can influence PC screening and detection.[94,111,114–117] For example, several studies have identified SNPs within or near KLK3 that can influence serum PSA concentrations in men without PC.[118–126] Similarly, the results of a recent GWAS documented that some of the PC-risk SNPs show strong associations with serum PSA levels.[94] Six SNPs in or near genes encoding telomerase reverse transcriptase (TERT; chromosome 5p15.33, SNP rs2736098), β-microseminoprotein (MSMB; chromosome 10q11, rs10993994), fibroblast growth factor receptor 2 (FGFR2; chromosome 10q26, rs10788160), T-box transcription factor (TBX3; chromosome 12q24, rs11067228), hepatocyte nuclear factor 1B (HNF1B; chromosome 17q12, rs4430796), and KLK3 (chromosome 19q13.33, rs17632542) seem to influence levels of PSA expression. Four of these SNPs (called PSA-SNPs) were found to be independently associated with higher serum PSA concentrations.[94]

Gudmundsson and colleagues[94] assessed whether the presence of the 4 PSA-SNPs could be used to genetically correct a man's measured serum PSA in an Icelandic cohort. These genetically corrected PSA values significantly improved the performance of PSA as a screening tool (area under the curve [AUC] 73.2%) compared with unadjusted values (AUC 70.9%); these results have since been replicated in an independent patient population.[127,128] Similarly, a prior study from the Baltimore Longitudinal Study of Aging showed that the risk of finding PC on biopsy differed based on genotype for PSA-associated SNPs.[115] Finally, it was shown in a cohort of men of European ancestry without documented PC that genetic correction for the presence of the 4 PSA-SNPs could potentially result in an 18% to 22% reduction in the number of potentially unnecessary biopsies (defined by those men whose measured serum PSA fell below a biopsy threshold after correction for the SNPs). In addition, genetic correction for the absence of the PSA-SNPs could result in a 3% reduction in potentially delayed biopsies, defined by those men whose measured serum PSA rose above a biopsy threshold after correction for the SNPs.[111] When genetic correction was applied to a cohort of African American men, the same PSA-SNPs yielded different results: genetic correction prevented no unnecessary biopsies, but could have been used to avoid delaying necessary biopsies in 30% of patients.[129] The racial differences in genetic correction are intriguing, as it is known that African American men are significantly more likely to be diagnosed with more advanced stage of disease and experience 2- to 3-fold greater PC-specific mortality than men of European ancestry.[96–99] Genetically corrected PSA levels in both European Americans and African Americans may allow physicians to more accurately gauge the risk of PC, and thus avoid delays in diagnosis and treatment.[130]

USEFULNESS OF COMMON GENOMIC VARIATION IN IDENTIFYING AGGRESSIVE DISEASE

An important issue in the PSA screening debate is that although PSA screening saves many lives, it also leads to the overtreatment of many indolent PC that would otherwise never harm patients.[8] As such, there is an urgent need to identify biomarkers that can help distinguish aggressive from indolent PC disease. Common genetic variants could provide useful biomarkers.

Although most common genetic variants identified to date are associated with PC risk, most of these studies involved cases with low-risk or intermediate-risk, organ-confined tumors.[21] Similarly, previous genetic studies that focused on PC aggressiveness have typically involved heterogeneous definitions of aggressive disease, and have often relied on clinical (as opposed to the more accurate surgical) grading and staging of tumors.[131–141] As such, there is debate as to whether any of the approximately 80 SNPs[72] associated with PC susceptibility are also associated with disease aggressiveness. Most PC-risk variants identified from GWAS have not been associated with higher Gleason grade or tumor stage,[60,76,142–145] suggesting that they may largely influence the risk of detecting or developing PC, but not necessarily of having aggressive disease. Moreover, there is little evidence for an association between the total number of GWAS PC-risk alleles carried by an individual and the prognosis of PC.[75] However, this possibility is not excluded. Despite the lack of previous studies focusing on disease aggressiveness, there is accumulating evidence that some PC SNPs truly are associated with aggressiveness.[133–135,139–141,146–150]

The first studies to evaluate associations with PC aggressiveness were linkage analyses, and more than 10 different genome-wide linkage studies of aggressive PC have been reported.[146,151–153] The initial studies were focused on associations with higher Gleason scores, and implicated regions at 5q31-33, 7q32, and 19q12-13.11 as harboring aggressive PC loci. Further fine-mapping studies of the 7q32 linkage region suggested that genetic variants in the KLRG2 (killer cell lectin-like receptor subfamily G member 2) gene may be associated with Gleason score at diagnosis. Additional studies have also identified 22q as a potential aggressiveness locus.[79,154–156] To date, the largest linkage study for aggressive PC, performed by the ICPCG, identified loci on chromosomes 6p22.3, 11q14.1-14.3, and 20p11.21-q11.21 as having an effect, with a more modest signal observed at 8q24.[157]

In addition to linkage analysis, the candidate gene approach has also recently been used to interrogate genes that have been putatively associated with aggressive or advanced PC disease.[158–168] For example, a recent study used a candidate gene approach to genotype variants within genes that have previously been associated with various aspects of PC biology, such as inflammation, steroid-hormone production and metabolism, DNA repair, and vitamin D activity.[147] The investigators interrogated almost 1000 SNPs in more than 150 different genes, and found SNPs in 5 different genes (*LEPR, RNASEL, IL4, CRY1,* and *ARVCF*) that showed associations with lethal PC. Now that these studies have implicated several interesting candidate genes, follow-up studies are necessary to validate these findings and to fully understand their contributions to inherited risk for more aggressive PC.

Several GWAS have approached the question of PC aggressiveness. For example, Xu and colleagues[140] and FitzGerald and colleagues[139] reported an SNP on chromosome 17p12 and another on 15q13 that were present at significantly greater frequencies in men with aggressive disease. Similarly, Bensen and colleagues[101] reported that an SNP on chromosome 3p12 was associated with PC aggressiveness in European American but not African American men. Moreover, the 8q24 region held 7 significant SNPs, of which 2 were associated with PC aggressiveness in African American but not European American men. Of the remaining 5 SNPs, 3 were associated with aggressiveness in African American men and 2 in European American men. Ahn and colleagues[141] performed an association analysis between a panel of 12 SNPs and PC metastasis and biochemical recurrence using the Cancer Genetic Markers of Susceptibility (CGEMS) database. Their results suggest that rs10993994 (chromosome 10q11; RR = 1.24), rs4242382 (chromosome 8q24; RR = 1.40), and rs6983267 (chromosome 8q24; RR = 0.67) were associated with metastatic PC. Similarly, Amin Al Olama and colleagues[134] conducted a meta-analysis involving a relatively large cohort of men aimed at determining whether SNPs were associated with adverse pathologic features. These investigators found a locus on chromosome 19 that was associated with aggressive disease, and another on chromosome 22 marginally associated with disease aggressiveness.

Bensen and colleagues[101] also reported that 3 SNPs in and around the *KLK3* gene on chromosome 19q13 were associated with PC aggressiveness.[94] For this subgroup, patients with lower PSA levels had more aggressive disease and higher Gleason scores. Other associations between Gleason grade and SNPs within the *KLK3* gene have been reported.[75,169] The minor alleles of these SNPs were associated with lower PSA levels, suggesting that carriers are less likely to

be diagnosed at an early stage through PSA screening.[94,170–172] Lindstrom and colleagues[173] reported that 2 SNPs located near *KLK3* were associated with PSA levels and Gleason grade. Similarly, Gudmundsson and colleagues[94] found that the *KLK3* association with PC was confined to cases diagnosed in the PSA era. Men with variants that increase PSA levels were more likely to undergo biopsy, but less likely to be diagnosed with PC and more likely to have early-stage disease at a younger age. Conversely, men with variants that decrease serum PSA levels were less likely to undergo biopsy but, when finally biopsied, were more likely to have PC and more advanced disease at an older age. Thus, *KLK3* variation might influence high-grade PC risk simply through its influence on PSA levels in a PC screening environment.

There is some debate about whether any of the newly identified rare variants in the *HOXB13* gene and on 8q24 are associated with adverse pathologic features or clinical outcomes. One study suggested that *HOXB13* gene mutations are associated with a higher Gleason score, as well as advanced stage of disease.[174] Similarly, a recent study evaluating *HOXB13* G84E mutation in more than 2440 hereditary PC families recruited by members of the ICPCG documented that more than one-third of *HOXB13* mutation carriers had a Gleason score of 7 or more, and more than one-quarter of these had non–organ-confined disease at diagnosis (tumor stage $\geq$T3). The mean age at diagnosis of *HOXB13* mutation carriers was younger (62.8 vs 64.4 years) than in more than 6000 PC patients without the mutation (P = .04).[175] Another study reported similar results: carriers of the mutation were diagnosed 1.26 years younger than noncarriers.[63] Similar analyses of the rs188140481[A] variant on 8q24 also show a marginal association with aggressive phenotypes (OR = 1.30; P = .08) and younger age of PC diagnosis (1.26 years).[63]

Thus, although it has become obvious that genetic factors influence overall PC susceptibility, the extent to which these genetic factors influence PC aggressiveness remains to be determined. To identify the true genetic variants associated with PC aggressiveness, studies enlisting appropriate patient cohorts (including large numbers of aggressive cases and large numbers of nonaggressive cases and controls) and using consistent definitions of aggressive disease must be performed. The results of these studies have the potential to provide major benefits in terms of identifying the most appropriate candidates (ie, those at risk for developing life-threatening disease) for PC screening.

USEFULNESS OF SOMATIC MARKERS IN SCREENING FOR AND DIAGNOSIS OF PROSTATE CANCER

Tumorigenesis is characterized by a progression of changes at the cellular, genetic, and epigenetic level that ultimately reprogram a cell to undergo uncontrolled cell division. It is possible that germ-line DNA variations contribute to PC tumorigenesis by making cells more susceptible to genetic changes and mutations. The resultant genetic changes that occur within the tumor (ie, somatic-level mutations) can also be characterized and used as potential biomarkers that help improve PC staging and treatment. In fact, many different assays that take advantage of somatic changes within prostate tumors are now commercially available (**Table 2**). For example, Myriad Genetics offers an assay (Prolaris) of prostate biopsy tissue that analyzes the expression of 31 different genes involved in cell-cycle proliferation as a way to examine for an increased likelihood of PC-specific mortality in men undergoing watchful waiting, as well as biochemical recurrence after radical surgery for PC.[176] Similarly, Genomic Health Inc offers Oncotype DX, Prostate, a test that determines the expression of 17 different genes involved in androgen signaling, cell organization, and proliferation, to predict upgrading or upstaging at the time of radical prostatectomy.[177] While many of these novel clinical tests are still under investigation, await validation, and are associated with proprietary information, they have potential to improve the diagnosis and management of PC.

Another recurring theme in this review is that advances in technology and decreases in cost have increased the ability to perform genetic sequencing studies and the potential to discover novel translocation events and mutations. As such, large efforts are currently being devoted toward studying the DNA landscape of PC tumors with particular emphasis on aggressive disease. As in many other human cancers, genomic alterations including mutations, insertions/deletions, translocations, inversions, gene fusions, and copy-number alterations (CNAs) have been identified in PC tumors.[178] Some of these genetic alterations are common across different prostate tumor specimens and are thus speculated to play a crucial role in tumorigenesis and progression. However, PC is considered to be a heterogeneous disease and, as such, various combinations of somatic-level genomic alterations have been identified among different tumors or even within the same tumor. This genetic heterogeneity is considered to be a key obstacle to distinguishing aggressive from indolent forms of PC.[179,180]

USEFULNESS OF DIFFERENCES IN TUMOR GENE EXPRESSION IN SCREENING FOR AND TREATMENT OF PROSTATE CANCER

PSA exists in 2 forms, free (unbound) and bound to α1-antichymotripsin. The percentage of free PSA (%fPSA) tends to increase with benign prostatic hyperplasia in comparison with PC.[181] A lower % fPSA is associated with increased PC risk, and studies have suggested that measuring %fPSA or complexed PSA adds to the diagnostic accuracy of PC.[182,183] Past studies have documented that a form of free PSA, called [-2] proenzyme PSA (p2PSA), is elevated in cancerous prostate tissue.[184,185] Beckman Coulter now offers a blood-based assay that takes advantage of p2PSA levels to aid in PC screening and treatment decisions. Specifically, Beckman Coulter has mathematically formulated a combination of the expression levels of total PSA, %fPSA, and p2PSA to calculate the Prostate Health Index (*phi*).[186–189] Several large, multi-institutional studies have demonstrated that the use of *phi* reduced the risk of unnecessary biopsies resulting from false-positive elevations in PSA, and was significantly better at identifying high-risk, potentially lethal prostate tumors, than the standard PSA test or the %fPSA alone.[190–192]

Prostate cancer gene 3 (PCA3; formerly referred to as DD3) is a noncoding RNA produced in the prostate.[193] It was shown to be overexpressed in 95% of prostate tumors, with a median 66-fold upregulation compared with adjacent noncancerous prostate tissue.[194] Given its high specificity and overexpression in PC tissue, a urine-based test was developed as a biomarker to aid in screening and detection (see **Table 2**). Testing for the biomarker involves collection of urine samples after a digital rectal examination is performed. Samples are centrifuged, and a PCA3 score is determined by comparing the levels of PCA3 mRNA with PSA mRNA.[193] Several studies have demonstrated that urinary PCA3 levels are significantly correlated with the percentage of men with biopsy-proven PC, and that it has reported sensitivities and specificities up to 76% and 90%, respectively.[195] Other research has suggested that PCA3 scores correlate with prostatectomy Gleason score and tumor volume,[196,197] although this is subject to debate.[198] However, this urine-based biomarker has the potential to add to current algorithms in identifying men who should be offered a repeat biopsy and/or who may harbor aggressive tumors. Of interest, several investigators are now evaluating whether PCA3 should be used in combination with other expression biomarkers such as *phi* or

Table 2
Several commercially available genetic assays based on somatic mutations within prostate cancer tumors

Proposed Utility	Test Name	Commercial Company	Sample	Measures	Web site
Distinguish between aggressive and nonaggressive prostate tumors	Prolaris	Myriad Genetics	Prostate biopsy tissue	31-gene expression panel involved in cell-cycle progression	http://www.myriad.com/treating-diseases/prostate-cancer/
	Oncotype Dx Prostate	Genomic Health, Inc	Prostate biopsy tissue	17-gene expression panel involved in stromal response, androgen signaling, cell organization, and proliferation	http://prostate-cancer.oncotypedx.com/en-US/Professional/IntroducingGPS/ValidationClinicalExperience.aspx http://prostate-cancer.oncotypedx.com/en-US/Professional/Resources/Bibliography
	ProstaVysion	Bostwick Laboratories	Prostate biopsy tissue	ERG gene fusion/translocation, Loss of PTEN	https://www.bostwicklaboratories.com/services/laboratory-services/urologic-pathology/ProstaVysion.aspx
Determine need for repeat biopsy after a negative prostate biopsy	Progensa PCA3	Gen-Probe (Hologic)	Urine	PCA3 gene expression	http://www.gen-probe.com/products-services/progensa-pca3
	ConfirmMDx	MDxHealth	Prostate biopsy tissue	Methylation of *GSTP1*, *APC*, *RASSF1* genes	http://www.mdxhealth.com/products-and-technology/products/confirmmdx-for-prostate-cancer
	Prostate Core Mitomic Test	Mitomics	Prostate biopsy tissue	Deletions of mitochondrial DNA	http://www.mitomicsinc.com/prostate-core-mitomic-test/
Determine metastasis after radical prostatectomy	Decipher	Genome Dx Bioscience	Prostate tissue	22 gene multipathway expression panel	http://www.genomedx.com/genomedxs-decipher-test-for-prostate-cancer-predicts-metastasis-impacts-treatment-decisions/

Adapted from Refs. [24,84,85,152,176,196,222–230]

TMPRSS2:ERG fusion (see later discussion). Preliminary results suggest that PCA3 and *phi* are superior to the other evaluated parameters (eg, PSA) in diagnostic accuracy for PC at the initial or repeat prostate biopsy.[186,199] Further prospective studies in larger populations are needed to confirm these results.

USEFULNESS OF COPY-NUMBER ALTERATIONS IN SCREENING FOR AND TREATMENT OF PROSTATE CANCER

CNAs are changes in the number of copies of specific regions of DNA that range in size from 1 kilobase to a complete chromosome arm, and mainly involve copy-number losses (deletions) or gains (amplifications). Current GWAS and sequencing studies of PC have revealed that CNAs are a major component of the landscape of the PC tumor genome.[179] Among the most common CNAs are amplifications of genomic regions of the 8q24 locus containing the *MYC* oncogene (20%–35%) as well as deletions of DNA sequences containing the tumor-suppressor genes, such as *NKX3-1* (8p21; 35%–70%), *PTEN* (10q23.31; 10%–40%), *CDKN1B* (12p13.1; 5%–40%), *RB1* (13q14.2; 25%–45%), and *TP53* (17p13.1; 20%–30%).[200] Because many of these regions reside in proximity or appear to interact through functional enhancers with many of the germline PC-risk SNPs, it is possible that germline variation may exert its influence by increasing susceptibility to somatic mutation. It is also noteworthy that the frequencies of many of these CNAs vary among different tumor samples, depending on the composition of cohorts, tumor grade, and degree of tumor-cell heterogeneity. For example, high-grade, metastatic prostate tumors typically contain more frequent CNAs than clinically localized PC.[201,202] In addition, some of the CNAs (eg, amplification of MYC or deletions of PTEN) have been associated with a worse clinical prognosis.[203–207] However, these results are inconsistent, which has limited their implementation into routine clinical practice. The reasons for these discrepancies may be related to facts such as chromosome gain or loss has not been consistently defined (eg, genetic deletion of the *PTEN* locus vs loss of protein expression), different outcomes are measured across studies (biochemical recurrence after local therapy vs PC-specific mortality in patients managed conservatively), and small numbers of patients are represented in each subgroup. However, taken together, future studies of CNAs may offer promise as a novel way to gauge PC aggressiveness.

USEFULNESS OF GENE TRANSLOCATIONS IN SCREENING FOR AND TREATMENT OF PROSTATE CANCER

Unlike many other solid tumors, PC contains a high frequency of gene fusions.[208] For example, it has been reported that the transmembrane protease, serine 2 v-ets erythroblastosis virus E26 oncogene homolog (avian) (TMPRSS2-ERG) translocation, is present in approximately half of all PC patients but is more common in men of European ancestry than in men of African ancestry.[209] To date, almost a dozen different gene fusions have been identified within PC tumors. In addition to *TMPRSS2-ERG* and other translocation events involving ETS family members, the solute carrier family 45 member 3-v-raf murine sarcoma viral oncogene homolog B1 (*SLC45A3-BRAF*) and epithelial splicing regulatory protein-1-v-raf-1 murine leukemia viral oncogene homolog 1 (*ESRP1-RAF1*) gene fusions also have been frequently documented in PC tumors.[210,211] However, the usefulness of these translocations in PC diagnosis and their impact on clinical outcome is controversial and still under investigation. For example, TMPRSS2-ERG has been implicated as both a negative and positive prognostic tumor marker.[212] However, in a large multi-institutional study it was shown that when TMPRSS-ERG levels are measured along with urinary PCA3 levels, they can be used to help predict whether a man has a positive biopsy or aggressive cancer (eg, increased Gleason grade disease).[199,213]

Recent technologies have now identified more than 5000 somatic mutations in prostate tumors, including recurrent translocations involving the cell-adhesion molecule CADM2 or the PTEN-interacting protein MAGI2, in addition to recurrent mutations of the Speckle-type POZ Protein (SPOP).[179,214,215] For localized tumors, the 12 most significantly mutated genes are *SPOP*, *FOXA1*, *TP53*, *PTEN*, *CDKN1B*, *MED12*, *THSD7B*, *SCN11A*, *NIPA2*, *PIK3CA*, *ZNF595*, and *C14orf49*. *SPOP* was the most commonly mutated gene in these tumors, with a frequency of 13%.[214] Of interest, no tumors with SPOP mutations carried ETS family gene rearrangements, but did show associations with deletions on chromosomes 5q21 and 6q21. Based on these observations, it was proposed that SPOP mutations may define a distinct molecular subtype of PC.[214] It is possible that these mutations and genetic alterations will prove to be advantageous in the clinical management of PC patients. In fact, novel therapeutics that directly target many of these genetic alterations (*ERG*, mutated *SPOP*, and so forth) in PC are currently under investigation. Future studies involving larger samples sizes and cancers at various stages of progression will allow for better definition of the genetic alterations in PC and how these events might alter clinical algorithms.

SUMMARY

With advances in genotyping and sequencing technologies at a fraction of the cost, continued discovery of novel germline and somatic genetic markers associated with disease initiation, progression, and response to treatment is anticipated in the future. Translation of these discoveries into routine clinical diagnostic tests and screening tools that provide personalized medicine should be possible. Ultimately prospective, large clinical trials involving multi-institutional collaborations will be required to validate the usefulness of these germline and somatic genetic markers in the management of PC. In the meantime, continued genetic studies that identify novel genetic variations in all forms of PC are critical to advancing our knowledge of the genetic basis of the disease.

ACKNOWLEDGMENTS

The authors would like to thank Katherine T. Sentell, Daniel Reinhardt, and Phillip R. Cooper for their help in the preparation of this article.

REFERENCES

1. Ferlay J, Shin HR, Bray F, et al. Estimates of worldwide burden of cancer in 2008: GLOBOCAN 2008. Int J Cancer 2010;127(12):2893–917.
2. Shin HR, Masuyer E, Ferlay J, et al. Cancer in Asia—incidence rates based on data in cancer incidence in five continents IX (1998-2002). Asian Pac J Cancer Prev 2010;11(Suppl 2):11–6.
3. Jemal A, Bray F, Center MM, et al. Global cancer statistics. CA Cancer J Clin 2011;61(2):69–90.
4. Bartsch G, Horninger W, Klocker H, et al. Tyrol prostate cancer demonstration project: early detection, treatment, outcome, incidence and mortality. BJU Int 2008;101(7):809–16.
5. Desireddi NV, Roehl KA, Loeb S, et al. Improved stage and grade-specific progression-free survival rates after radical prostatectomy in the PSA era. Urology 2007;70(5):950–5.
6. Amling CL. Prostate-specific antigen and detection of prostate cancer: What have we learned and what should we recommend for screening? Curr Treat Options Oncol 2006;7(5):337–45.
7. Trinchieri A, Moretti R. Trends in prostate cancer epidemiology in the year 2000. Arch Ital Urol Androl 2005;77(3):164–6.
8. Loeb S, Catalona WJ. Prostate-specific antigen screening: pro. Curr Opin Urol 2010;20(3):185–8.
9. Sanda MG, Dunn RL, Michalski J, et al. Quality of life and satisfaction with outcome among prostate-cancer survivors. N Engl J Med 2008; 358(12):1250–61.
10. Wilt TJ, Brawer MK, Jones KM, et al. Radical prostatectomy versus observation for localized prostate cancer. N Engl J Med 2012;367(3):203–13.
11. Ficarra V, Novara G, Rosen RC, et al. Systematic review and meta-analysis of studies reporting urinary continence recovery after robot-assisted radical prostatectomy. Eur Urol 2012;62(3):405–17.
12. Carter BS, Beaty TH, Steinberg GD, et al. Mendelian inheritance of familial prostate cancer. Proc Natl Acad Sci U S A 1992;89(8):3367–71.
13. Eeles RA. Genetic predisposition to prostate cancer. Prostate Cancer Prostatic Dis 1999;2(1):9–15.
14. Edwards SM, Eeles RA. Unravelling the genetics of prostate cancer. Am J Med Genet C Semin Med Genet 2004;129C(1):65–73.
15. Lichtenstein P, Holm NV, Verkasalo PK, et al. Environmental and heritable factors in the causation of cancer—analyses of cohorts of twins from Sweden, Denmark, and Finland. N Engl J Med 2000; 343(2):78–85.
16. Gronberg H, Wiklund F, Damber JE. Age specific risks of familial prostate carcinoma: a basis for screening recommendations in high risk populations. Cancer 1999;86(3):477–83.
17. Zeegers MP, Jellema A, Ostrer H. Empiric risk of prostate carcinoma for relatives of patients with prostate carcinoma: a meta-analysis. Cancer 2003;97(8):1894–903.
18. Bratt O. Hereditary prostate cancer: clinical aspects. J Urol 2002;168(3):906–13.
19. Zuhlke KA, Johnson AM, Okoth LA, et al. Identification of a novel NBN truncating mutation in a family with hereditary prostate cancer. Fam Cancer 2012; 11(4):595–600.
20. Isaacs WB. Inherited susceptibility for aggressive prostate cancer. Asian J Androl 2012;14(3):415–8.
21. Catalona WJ, Bailey-Wilson JE, Camp NJ, et al. National Cancer Institute prostate cancer genetics workshop. Cancer Res 2011;71(10):3442–6.
22. Choudhury AD, Eeles R, Freedland SJ, et al. The role of genetic markers in the management of prostate cancer. Eur Urol 2012;62(4):577–87.
23. Schaid DJ. The complex genetic epidemiology of prostate cancer. Hum Mol Genet 2004;13(Spec No 1):R103–21.
24. Xu J, Dimitrov L, Chang BL, et al. A combined genomewide linkage scan of 1,233 families for prostate cancer-susceptibility genes conducted by the international consortium for prostate cancer genetics. Am J Hum Genet 2005;77(2):219–29.
25. The Breast Cancer Linkage Consortium. Cancer risks in BRCA2 mutation carriers. J Natl Cancer Inst 1999;91(15):1310–6.

26. Castro E, Eeles R. The role of BRCA1 and BRCA2 in prostate cancer. Asian J Androl 2012;14(3): 409–14.

27. Bancroft EK, Page EC, Castro E, et al. Targeted Prostate Cancer Screening in BRCA1 and BRCA2 Mutation Carriers: Results from the Initial Screening Round of the IMPACT Study. Eur Urol 2014. [Epub ahead of Print].

28. Sundararajan S, Ahmed A, Goodman OB Jr. The relevance of BRCA genetics to prostate cancer pathogenesis and treatment. Clin Adv Hematol Oncol 2011;9(10):748–55.

29. Gudmundsdottir K, Ashworth A. The roles of BRCA1 and BRCA2 and associated proteins in the maintenance of genomic stability. Oncogene 2006;25(43):5864–74.

30. Boulton SJ. Cellular functions of the BRCA tumour-suppressor proteins. Biochem Soc Trans 2006; 34(Pt 5):633–45.

31. Turner N, Tutt A, Ashworth A. Hallmarks of 'BRCA-ness' in sporadic cancers. Nat Rev Cancer 2004; 4(10):814–9.

32. Agalliu I, Karlins E, Kwon EM, et al. Rare germline mutations in the BRCA2 gene are associated with early-onset prostate cancer. Br J Cancer 2007; 97(6):826–31.

33. Kote-Jarai Z, Leongamornlert D, Saunders E, et al. BRCA2 is a moderate penetrance gene contributing to young-onset prostate cancer: implications for genetic testing in prostate cancer patients. Br J Cancer 2011;105(8):1230–4.

34. Whittemore AS, Gong G, Itnyre J. Prevalence and contribution of BRCA1 mutations in breast cancer and ovarian cancer: results from three U.S. population-based case-control studies of ovarian cancer. Am J Hum Genet 1997;60(3):496–504.

35. Risch HA, McLaughlin JR, Cole DE, et al. Population BRCA1 and BRCA2 mutation frequencies and cancer penetrances: a kin-cohort study in Ontario, Canada. J Natl Cancer Inst 2006;98(23): 1694–706.

36. Roa BB, Boyd AA, Volcik K, et al. Ashkenazi Jewish population frequencies for common mutations in BRCA1 and BRCA2. Nat Genet 1996;14(2): 185–7.

37. Oddoux C, Struewing JP, Clayton CM, et al. The carrier frequency of the BRCA2 6174delT mutation among Ashkenazi Jewish individuals is approximately 1%. Nat Genet 1996;14(2):188–90.

38. Vazina A, Baniel J, Yaacobi Y, et al. The rate of the founder Jewish mutations in BRCA1 and BRCA2 in prostate cancer patients in Israel. Br J Cancer 2000;83(4):463–6.

39. Struewing JP, Hartge P, Wacholder S, et al. The risk of cancer associated with specific mutations of BRCA1 and BRCA2 among Ashkenazi Jews. N Engl J Med 1997;336(20):1401–8.

40. Tryggvadottir L, Vidarsdottir L, Thorgeirsson T, et al. Prostate cancer progression and survival in BRCA2 mutation carriers. J Natl Cancer Inst 2007;99(12):929–35.

41. Thorne H, Willems AJ, Niedermayr E, et al. Decreased prostate cancer-specific survival of men with BRCA2 mutations from multiple breast cancer families. Cancer Prev Res (Phila) 2011;4(7):1002–10.

42. Edwards SM, Evans DG, Hope Q, et al. Prostate cancer in BRCA2 germline mutation carriers is associated with poorer prognosis. Br J Cancer 2010;103(6):918–24.

43. Narod SA, Neuhausen S, Vichodez G, et al. Rapid progression of prostate cancer in men with a BRCA2 mutation. Br J Cancer 2008;99(2):371–4.

44. Gallagher DJ, Gaudet MM, Pal P, et al. Germline BRCA mutations denote a clinicopathologic subset of prostate cancer. Clin Cancer Res 2010;16(7): 2115–21.

45. Yang D, Khan S, Sun Y, et al. Association of BRCA1 and BRCA2 mutations with survival, chemotherapy sensitivity, and gene mutator phenotype in patients with ovarian cancer. JAMA 2011;306(14):1557–65.

46. Fong PC, Boss DS, Yap TA, et al. Inhibition of poly(ADP-ribose) polymerase in tumors from BRCA mutation carriers. N Engl J Med 2009; 361(2):123–34.

47. Fong PC, Yap TA, Boss DS, et al. Poly(ADP)-ribose polymerase inhibition: frequent durable responses in BRCA carrier ovarian cancer correlating with platinum-free interval. J Clin Oncol 2010;28(15): 2512–9.

48. Gallagher DJ, Cronin AM, Milowsky MI, et al. Germline BRCA mutation does not prevent response to taxane-based therapy for the treatment of castration-resistant prostate cancer. BJU Int 2012; 109(5):713–9.

49. Stoffel E, Mukherjee B, Raymond VM, et al. Calculation of risk of colorectal and endometrial cancer among patients with Lynch syndrome. Gastroenterology 2009;137(5):1621–7.

50. Aarnio M, Mecklin JP, Aaltonen LA, et al. Life-time risk of different cancers in hereditary non-polyposis colorectal cancer (HNPCC) syndrome. Int J Cancer 1995;64(6):430–3.

51. Raymond VM, Mukherjee B, Wang F, et al. Elevated risk of prostate cancer among men with lynch syndrome. J Clin Oncol 2013;31(14):1713–8.

52. Bauer CM, Ray AM, Halstead-Nussloch BA, et al. Hereditary prostate cancer as a feature of Lynch syndrome. Fam Cancer 2011;10(1):37–42.

53. da Silva FC, de Oliveira LP, Santos EM, et al. Frequency of extracolonic tumors in Brazilian families with Lynch syndrome: analysis of a hereditary colorectal cancer institutional registry. Fam Cancer 2010;9(4):563–70.

54. Goecke T, Schulmann K, Engel C, et al. Genotype-phenotype comparison of German MLH1 and MSH2 mutation carriers clinically affected with Lynch syndrome: a report by the German HNPCC Consortium. J Clin Oncol 2006;24(26): 4285–92.

55. Scott RJ, McPhillips M, Meldrum CJ, et al. Hereditary nonpolyposis colorectal cancer in 95 families: differences and similarities between mutation-positive and mutation-negative kindreds. Am J Hum Genet 2001;68(1):118–27.

56. Kruglyak L, Nickerson DA. Variation is the spice of life. Nat Genet 2001;27(3):234–6.

57. Marian AJ. Molecular genetic studies of complex phenotypes. Transl Res 2012;159(2):64–79.

58. Verma RS, Manikal M, Conte RA, et al. Chromosomal basis of adenocarcinoma of the prostate. Cancer Invest 1999;17(6):441–7.

59. Bova GS, Isaacs WB. Review of allelic loss and gain in prostate cancer. World J Urol 1996;14(5):338–46.

60. Freedman ML, Haiman CA, Patterson N, et al. Admixture mapping identifies 8q24 as a prostate cancer risk locus in African-American men. Proc Natl Acad Sci U S A 2006;103(38):14068–73.

61. Amundadottir LT, Sulem P, Gudmundsson J, et al. A common variant associated with prostate cancer in European and African populations. Nat Genet 2006;38(6):652–8.

62. Al Olama AA, Kote-Jarai Z, Giles GG, et al. Multiple loci on 8q24 associated with prostate cancer susceptibility. Nat Genet 2009;41(10):1058–60.

63. Gudmundsson J, Sulem P, Gudbjartsson DF, et al. A study based on whole-genome sequencing yields a rare variant at 8q24 associated with prostate cancer. Nat Genet 2012;44(12):1326–9.

64. Robbins C, Torres JB, Hooker S, et al. Confirmation study of prostate cancer risk variants at 8q24 in African Americans identifies a novel risk locus. Genome Res 2007;17(12):1717–22.

65. Ellwood-Yen K, Graeber TG, Wongvipat J, et al. Myc-driven murine prostate cancer shares molecular features with human prostate tumors. Cancer Cell 2003;4(3):223–38.

66. Yeager M, Orr N, Hayes RB, et al. Genome-wide association study of prostate cancer identifies a second risk locus at 8q24. Nat Genet 2007;39(5): 645–9.

67. Jia L, Landan G, Pomerantz M, et al. Functional enhancers at the gene-poor 8q24 cancer-linked locus. PLoS Genet 2009;5(8):e1000597.

68. Ahmadiyeh N, Pomerantz MM, Grisanzio C, et al. 8q24 prostate, breast, and colon cancer risk loci show tissue-specific long-range interaction with MYC. Proc Natl Acad Sci U S A 2010;107(21): 9742–6.

69. Pomerantz MM, Beckwith CA, Regan MM, et al. Evaluation of the 8q24 prostate cancer risk locus and MYC expression. Cancer Res 2009;69(13): 5568–74.

70. Tuupanen S, Turunen M, Lehtonen R, et al. The common colorectal cancer predisposition SNP rs6983267 at chromosome 8q24 confers potential to enhanced Wnt signaling. Nat Genet 2009; 41(8):885–90.

71. Meyer KB, Maia AT, O'Reilly M, et al. A functional variant at a prostate cancer predisposition locus at 8q24 is associated with PVT1 expression. PLoS Genet 2011;7(7):e1002165.

72. Eeles RA, Olama AA, Benlloch S, et al. Identification of 23 new prostate cancer susceptibility loci using the iCOGS custom genotyping array. Nat Genet 2013;45(4):385–91, 391.e1–2.

73. Kote-Jarai Z, Saunders EJ, Leongamornlert DA, et al. Fine-mapping identifies multiple prostate cancer risk loci at 5p15, one of which associates with TERT expression. Hum Mol Genet 2013;22(12):2520–8.

74. Foulkes WD. Inherited susceptibility to common cancers. N Engl J Med 2008;359(20):2143–53.

75. Kader AK, Sun J, Isaacs SD, et al. Individual and cumulative effect of prostate cancer risk-associated variants on clinicopathologic variables in 5,895 prostate cancer patients. Prostate 2009; 69(11):1195–205.

76. Wiklund FE, Adami HO, Zheng SL, et al. Established prostate cancer susceptibility variants are not associated with disease outcome. Cancer Epidemiol Biomarkers Prev 2009;18(5):1659–62.

77. Sun J, Chang BL, Isaacs SD, et al. Cumulative effect of five genetic variants on prostate cancer risk in multiple study populations. Prostate 2008; 68(12):1257–62.

78. Zheng SL, Sun J, Wiklund F, et al. Cumulative association of five genetic variants with prostate cancer. N Engl J Med 2008;358(9):910–9.

79. Lange EM, Gillanders EM, Davis CC, et al. Genome-wide scan for prostate cancer susceptibility genes using families from the University of Michigan prostate cancer genetics project finds evidence for linkage on chromosome 17 near BRCA1. Prostate 2003;57(4):326–34.

80. Gillanders EM, Xu J, Chang BL, et al. Combined genome-wide scan for prostate cancer susceptibility genes. J Natl Cancer Inst 2004;96(16):1240–7.

81. Ewing CM, Ray AM, Lange EM, et al. Germline mutations in HOXB13 and prostate-cancer risk. N Engl J Med 2012;366(2):141–9.

82. Breyer JP, Avritt TG, McReynolds KM, et al. Confirmation of the HOXB13 G84E germline mutation in familial prostate cancer. Cancer Epidemiol Biomarkers Prev 2012;21(8):1348–53.

83. Akbari MR, Trachtenberg J, Lee J, et al. Association between germline HOXB13 G84E mutation and risk of prostate cancer. J Natl Cancer Inst 2012;104(16):1260–2.

84. Karlsson R, Aly M, Clements M, et al. A population-based assessment of germline HOXB13 G84E mutation and prostate cancer risk. Eur Urol 2014; 65(1):169–76.

85. Lin X, Qu L, Chen Z, et al. A novel germline mutation in HOXB13 is associated with prostate cancer risk in Chinese men. Prostate 2013;73(2):169–75.

86. Laitinen VH, Wahlfors T, Saaristo L, et al. HOXB13 G84E mutation in Finland: population-based analysis of prostate, breast, and colorectal cancer risk. Cancer Epidemiol Biomarkers Prev 2013; 22(3):452–60.

87. Xu J, Sun J, Kader AK, et al. Estimation of absolute risk for prostate cancer using genetic markers and family history. Prostate 2009;69(14):1565–72.

88. Helfand BT, Kan D, Modi P, et al. Prostate cancer risk alleles significantly improve disease detection and are associated with aggressive features in patients with a "normal" prostate specific antigen and digital rectal examination. Prostate 2011;71(4): 394–402.

89. Wang M, Liu F, Hsing AW, et al. Replication and cumulative effects of GWAS-identified genetic variations for prostate cancer in Asians: a case-control study in the ChinaPCa consortium. Carcinogenesis 2012;33(2):356–60.

90. Chen M, Huang YC, Yang S, et al. Common variants at 8q24 are associated with prostate cancer risk in Taiwanese men. Prostate 2010;70(5):502–7.

91. Helfand BT, Loeb S, Kan D, et al. Number of prostate cancer risk alleles may identify possibly 'insignificant' disease. BJU Int 2010;106(11):1602–6.

92. Spitz MR, Etzel CJ, Dong Q, et al. An expanded risk prediction model for lung cancer. Cancer Prev Res (Phila) 2008;1(4):250–4.

93. Barlow WE, White E, Ballard-Barbash R, et al. Prospective breast cancer risk prediction model for women undergoing screening mammography. J Natl Cancer Inst 2006;98(17):1204–14.

94. Gudmundsson J, Besenbacher S, Sulem P, et al. Genetic correction of PSA values using sequence variants associated with PSA levels. Sci Transl Med 2010;2(62):62ra92.

95. Aly M, Wiklund F, Xu J, et al. Polygenic risk score improves prostate cancer risk prediction: results from the Stockholm-1 cohort study. Eur Urol 2011; 60(1):21–8.

96. Odedina FT, Akinremi TO, Chinegwundoh F, et al. Prostate cancer disparities in Black men of African descent: a comparative literature review of prostate cancer burden among Black men in the United States, Caribbean, United Kingdom, and West Africa. Infect Agent Cancer 2009;4(Suppl 1):S2.

97. Williams H, Powell IJ. Epidemiology, pathology, and genetics of prostate cancer among African Americans compared with other ethnicities. Methods Mol Biol 2009;472:439–53.

98. Powell IJ, Banerjee M, Bianco FJ, et al. The effect of race/ethnicity on prostate cancer treatment outcome is conditional: a review of Wayne State University data. J Urol 2004;171(4):1508–12.

99. Ishak MB, Giri VN. A systematic review of replication studies of prostate cancer susceptibility genetic variants in high-risk men originally identified from genome-wide association studies. Cancer Epidemiol Biomarkers Prev 2011;20(8):1599–610.

100. Okobia MN, Zmuda JM, Ferrell RE, et al. Chromosome 8q24 variants are associated with prostate cancer risk in a high risk population of African ancestry. Prostate 2011;71(10):1054–63.

101. Bensen JT, Xu Z, Smith GJ, et al. Genetic polymorphism and prostate cancer aggressiveness: a case-only study of 1,536 GWAS and candidate SNPs in African-Americans and European-Americans. Prostate 2013;73(1):11–22.

102. Haiman CA, Chen GK, Blot WJ, et al. Characterizing genetic risk at known prostate cancer susceptibility loci in African Americans. PLoS Genet 2011;7(5):e1001387.

103. Haiman CA, Chen GK, Blot WJ, et al. Genome-wide association study of prostate cancer in men of African ancestry identifies a susceptibility locus at 17q21. Nat Genet 2011;43(6):570–3.

104. Xu Z, Bensen JT, Smith GJ, et al. GWAS SNP Replication among African American and European American men in the North Carolina-Louisiana prostate cancer project (PCaP). Prostate 2011; 71(8):881–91.

105. Whitman EJ, Pomerantz M, Chen Y, et al. Prostate cancer risk allele specific for African descent associates with pathologic stage at prostatectomy. Cancer Epidemiol Biomarkers Prev 2010;19(1):1–8.

106. Hooker S, Hernandez W, Chen H, et al. Replication of prostate cancer risk loci on 8q24, 11q13, 17q12, 19q33, and Xp11 in African Americans. Prostate 2010;70(3):270–5.

107. Xu J, Kibel AS, Hu JJ, et al. Prostate cancer risk associated loci in African Americans. Cancer Epidemiol Biomarkers Prev 2009;18(7):2145–9.

108. Chang BL, Spangler E, Gallagher S, et al. Validation of genome-wide prostate cancer associations in men of African descent. Cancer Epidemiol Biomarkers Prev 2011;20(1):23–32.

109. Zeigler-Johnson CM, Rennert H, Mittal RD, et al. Evaluation of prostate cancer characteristics in four populations worldwide. Can J Urol 2008; 15(3):4056–64.

110. Djavan B, Eckersberger E, Finkelstein J, et al. Prostate-specific antigen testing and prostate cancer screening. Prim Care 2010;37(3):441–59, vii.

111. Helfand BT, Loeb S, Hu Q, et al. Personalized prostate specific antigen testing using genetic variants may reduce unnecessary prostate biopsies. J Urol 2013;189(5):1697–701.

112. Bansal A, Murray DK, Wu JT, et al. Heritability of prostate-specific antigen and relationship with zonal prostate volumes in aging twins. J Clin Endocrinol Metab 2000;85(3):1272–6.

113. Pilia G, Chen WM, Scuteri A, et al. Heritability of cardiovascular and personality traits in 6,148 Sardinians. PLoS Genet 2006;2(8):e132.

114. Loeb S. Germline sequence variants and prostate-specific antigen interpretation. Clin Chem 2011; 57(5):662–3.

115. Loeb S, Carter HB, Walsh PC, et al. Single nucleotide polymorphisms and the likelihood of prostate cancer at a given prostate specific antigen level. J Urol 2009;182(1):101–4 [discussion: 105].

116. Guy M, Kote-Jarai Z, Giles GG, et al. Identification of new genetic risk factors for prostate cancer. Asian J Androl 2009;11(1):49–55.

117. Nam RK, Zhang WW, Klotz LH, et al. Variants of the hK2 protein gene (KLK2) are associated with serum hK2 levels and predict the presence of prostate cancer at biopsy. Clin Cancer Res 2006; 12(21):6452–8.

118. Lose F, Batra J, O'Mara T, et al. Common variation in Kallikrein genes KLK5, KLK6, KLK12, and KLK13 and risk of prostate cancer and tumor aggressiveness. Urol Oncol 2011;31(5):635–43.

119. Pomerantz MM, Werner L, Xie W, et al. Association of prostate cancer risk Loci with disease aggressiveness and prostate cancer-specific mortality. Cancer Prev Res (Phila) 2011;4(5): 719–28.

120. Kohli M, Rothberg PG, Feng C, et al. Exploratory study of a KLK2 polymorphism as a prognostic marker in prostate cancer. Cancer Biomark 2010; 7(2):101–8.

121. Cheng I, Plummer SJ, Neslund-Dudas C, et al. Prostate cancer susceptibility variants confer increased risk of disease progression. Cancer Epidemiol Biomarkers Prev 2010;19(9):2124–32.

122. Cramer SD, Sun J, Zheng SL, et al. Association of prostate-specific antigen promoter genotype with clinical and histopathologic features of prostate cancer. Cancer Epidemiol Biomarkers Prev 2008; 17(9):2451–7.

123. Pal P, Xi H, Sun G, et al. Tagging SNPs in the kallikrein genes 3 and 2 on 19q13 and their associations with prostate cancer in men of European origin. Hum Genet 2007;122(3–4):251–9.

124. Lu X, Zhao W, Huang J, et al. Common variation in KLKB1 and essential hypertension risk: tagging-SNP haplotype analysis in a case-control study. Hum Genet 2007;121(3–4):327–35.

125. Cramer SD, Chang BL, Rao A, et al. Association between genetic polymorphisms in the prostate-specific antigen gene promoter and serum prostate-specific antigen levels. J Natl Cancer Inst 2003;95(14):1044–53.

126. Parikh H, Wang Z, Pettigrew KA, et al. Fine mapping the KLK3 locus on chromosome 19q13.33 associated with prostate cancer susceptibility and PSA levels. Hum Genet 2011;129(6):675–85.

127. Vickers A, Cronin A, Roobol M, et al. Reducing unnecessary biopsy during prostate cancer screening using a four-kallikrein panel: an independent replication. J Clin Oncol 2010;28(15): 2493–8.

128. Vickers AJ, Cronin AM, Roobol MJ, et al. A four-kallikrein panel predicts prostate cancer in men with recent screening: data from the European Randomized Study of Screening for Prostate Cancer, Rotterdam. Clin Cancer Res 2010;16(12): 3232–9.

129. Donin N, Loeb S, Cooper PR, et al. Genetically adjusted prostate-specific antigen values may prevent delayed biopsies in African-American men. BJU Int, in press.

130. Scardino PT. Prostate cancer: improving PSA testing by adjusting for genetic background. Nat Rev Urol 2013;10(4):190–2.

131. Kwon EM, Salinas CA, Kolb S, et al. Genetic polymorphisms in inflammation pathway genes and prostate cancer risk. Cancer Epidemiol Biomarkers Prev 2011;20(5):923–33.

132. Camp NJ, Farnham JM, Wong J, et al. Replication of the 10q11 and Xp11 prostate cancer risk variants: results from a Utah pedigree-based study. Cancer Epidemiol Biomarkers Prev 2009;18(4): 1290–4.

133. Lu L, Cancel-Tassin G, Valeri A, et al. Chromosomes 4 and 8 implicated in a genome wide SNP linkage scan of 762 prostate cancer families collected by the ICPCG. Prostate 2012;72(4): 410–26.

134. Amin Al Olama A, Kote-Jarai Z, Schumacher FR, et al. A meta-analysis of genome-wide association studies to identify prostate cancer susceptibility loci associated with aggressive and non-aggressive disease. Hum Mol Genet 2013;22(2): 408–15.

135. Penney KL, Pyne S, Schumacher FR, et al. Genome-wide association study of prostate cancer mortality. Cancer Epidemiol Biomarkers Prev 2010; 19(11):2869–76.

136. Pal P, Xi H, Guha S, et al. Common variants in 8q24 are associated with risk for prostate cancer and tumor aggressiveness in men of European ancestry. Prostate 2009;69(14):1548–56.

137. Gudmundsson J, Sulem P, Rafnar T, et al. Common sequence variants on 2p15 and Xp11.22 confer susceptibility to prostate cancer. Nat Genet 2008; 40(3):281–3.

138. Duggan D, Zheng SL, Knowlton M, et al. Two genome-wide association studies of aggressive prostate cancer implicate putative prostate tumor

Prostate Health Index using WHO calibration. J Urol 2013;189(5):1702–6.

193. Hessels D, Klein Gunnewiek JM, van Oort I, et al. DD3(PCA3)-based molecular urine analysis for the diagnosis of prostate cancer. Eur Urol 2003; 44(1):8–15 [discussion: 15–6].

194. de Kok JB, Verhaegh GW, Roelofs RW, et al. DD3(PCA3), a very sensitive and specific marker to detect prostate tumors. Cancer Res 2002; 62(9):2695–8.

195. Deras IL, Aubin SM, Blase A, et al. PCA3: a molecular urine assay for predicting prostate biopsy outcome. J Urol 2008;179(4):1587–92.

196. Nakanishi H, Groskopf J, Fritsche HA, et al. PCA3 molecular urine assay correlates with prostate cancer tumor volume: implication in selecting candidates for active surveillance. J Urol 2008;179(5): 1804–9 [discussion: 1809–10].

197. Lin DW, Newcomb LF, Brown EC, et al. Urinary TMPRSS2:ERG and PCA3 in an active surveillance cohort: results from a baseline analysis in the Canary Prostate Active Surveillance Study. Clin Cancer Res 2013;19(9):2442–50.

198. Whitman EJ, Groskopf J, Ali A, et al. PCA3 score before radical prostatectomy predicts extracapsular extension and tumor volume. J Urol 2008; 180(5):1975–8 [discussion 1978–9].

199. Stephan C, Jung K, Semjonow A, et al. Comparative assessment of urinary prostate cancer antigen 3 and TMPRSS2:ERG gene fusion with the serum [-2]proprostate-specific antigen-based prostate health index for detection of prostate cancer. Clin Chem 2013;59(1):280–8.

200. Liu W, Xie CC, Zhu Y, et al. Homozygous deletions and recurrent amplifications implicate new genes involved in prostate cancer. Neoplasia 2008; 10(8):897–907.

201. Sun J, Liu W, Adams TS, et al. DNA copy number alterations in prostate cancers: a combined analysis of published CGH studies. Prostate 2007; 67(7):692–700.

202. Taylor BS, Schultz N, Hieronymus H, et al. Integrative genomic profiling of human prostate cancer. Cancer Cell 2010;18(1):11–22.

203. Nickerson ML, Im KM, Misner KJ, et al. Somatic alterations contributing to metastasis of a castration-resistant prostate cancer. Hum Mutat 2013;34(9): 1231–41.

204. Liu W, Xie CC, Thomas CY, et al. Genetic markers associated with early cancer-specific mortality following prostatectomy. Cancer 2013;119(13):2405–12.

205. Dean M, Lou H. Genetics and genomics of prostate cancer. Asian J Androl 2013;15(3):309–13.

206. Zafarana G, Ishkanian AS, Malloff CA, et al. Copy number alterations of c-MYC and PTEN are prognostic factors for relapse after prostate cancer radiotherapy. Cancer 2012;118(16):4053–62.

207. Cheng I, Levin AM, Tai YC, et al. Copy number alterations in prostate tumors and disease aggressiveness. Genes Chromosomes Cancer 2012; 51(1):66–76.

208. Kumar-Sinha C, Tomlins SA, Chinnaiyan AM. Recurrent gene fusions in prostate cancer. Nat Rev Cancer 2008;8(7):497–511.

209. Tomlins SA, Rhodes DR, Perner S, et al. Recurrent fusion of TMPRSS2 and ETS transcription factor genes in prostate cancer. Science 2005;310(5748): 644–8.

210. Palanisamy N, Ateeq B, Kalyana-Sundaram S, et al. Rearrangements of the RAF kinase pathway in prostate cancer, gastric cancer and melanoma. Nat Med 2010;16(7):793–8.

211. Kollermann J, Albrecht H, Schlomm T, et al. Activating BRAF gene mutations are uncommon in hormone refractory prostate cancer in Caucasian patients. Oncol Lett 2010;1(4):729–32.

212. Tomlins SA, Bjartell A, Chinnaiyan AM, et al. ETS gene fusions in prostate cancer: from discovery to daily clinical practice. Eur Urol 2009;56(2):275–86.

213. Tomlins SA, Aubin SM, Siddiqui J, et al. Urine TMPRSS2:ERG fusion transcript stratifies prostate cancer risk in men with elevated serum PSA. Sci Transl Med 2011;3(94):94ra72.

214. Barbieri CE, Baca SC, Lawrence MS, et al. Exome sequencing identifies recurrent SPOP, FOXA1 and MED12 mutations in prostate cancer. Nat Genet 2012;44(6):685–9.

215. Grasso CS, Wu YM, Robinson DR, et al. The mutational landscape of lethal castration-resistant prostate cancer. Nature 2012;487(7406):239–43.

216. Eeles RA, Kote-Jarai Z, Al Olama AA, et al. Identification of seven new prostate cancer susceptibility loci through a genome-wide association study. Nat Genet 2009;41(10):1116–21.

217. Gudmundsson J, Sulem P, Manolescu A, et al. Genome-wide association study identifies a second prostate cancer susceptibility variant at 8q24. Nat Genet 2007;39(5):631–7.

218. Gudmundsson J, Sulem P, Steinthorsdottir V, et al. Two variants on chromosome 17 confer prostate cancer risk, and the one in TCF2 protects against type 2 diabetes. Nat Genet 2007;39(8):977–83.

219. Kote-Jarai Z, Olama AA, Giles GG, et al. Seven prostate cancer susceptibility loci identified by a multi-stage genome-wide association study. Nat Genet 2011;43(8):785–91.

220. Schumacher FR, Berndt SI, Siddiq A, et al. Genome-wide association study identifies new prostate cancer susceptibility loci. Hum Mol Genet 2011;20(19):3867–75.

221. Thomas G, Jacobs KB, Yeager M, et al. Multiple loci identified in a genome-wide association study of prostate cancer. Nat Genet 2008;40(3): 310–5.

222. Cuzick J, Swanson GP, Fisher G, et al. Prognostic value of an RNA expression signature derived from cell cycle proliferation genes in patients with prostate cancer: a retrospective study. Lancet Oncol 2011;12(3):245–55.

223. Cuzick J, Berney DM, Fisher G, et al. Prognostic value of a cell cycle progression signature for prostate cancer death in a conservatively managed needle biopsy cohort. Br J Cancer 2012;106(6): 1095–9.

224. Bussemakers MJ, van Bokhoven A, Verhaegh GW, et al. DD3: a new prostate-specific gene, highly overexpressed in prostate cancer. Cancer Res 1999;59(23):5975–9.

225. de la Taille A. Progensa PCA3 test for prostate cancer detection. Expert Rev Mol Diagn 2007;7(5): 491–7.

226. Kirby R. PCA3 improves diagnosis of prostate cancer. Practitioner 2007;251(1690):18, 21, 23.

227. Stewart GD, Van Neste L, Delvenne P, et al. Clinical utility of an epigenetic assay to detect occult prostate cancer in histopathologically negative biopsies: results of the MATLOC study. J Urol 2013;189(3):1110–6.

228. Trock BJ, Brotzman MJ, Mangold LA, et al. Evaluation of GSTP1 and APC methylation as indicators for repeat biopsy in a high-risk cohort of men with negative initial prostate biopsies. BJU Int 2012; 110(1):56–62.

229. Robinson K, Creed J, Reguly B, et al. Accurate prediction of repeat prostate biopsy outcomes by a mitochondrial DNA deletion assay. Prostate Cancer Prostatic Dis 2010;13(2):126–31.

230. Badani K, Thompson DJ, Buerki C, et al. Impact of a genomic classifier of metastatic risk on postoperative treatment recommendations for prostate cancer patients: a report from the DECIDE study group. Oncotarget 2013;4(4):600–9.

Optimization of Prostate Biopsy
Review of Technique and Complications

Marc A. Bjurlin, DO, James S. Wysock, MD, MSCI,
Samir S. Taneja, MD*

KEYWORDS

- Prostate needle biopsy • Magnetic resonance imaging • Biopsy core number
- Quinolone-reistant infection

KEY POINTS

- A 12-core systematic biopsy that incorporates apical and far-lateral cores in the template distribution allows maximal cancer detection and avoidance of a repeat biopsy, while minimizing the detection of insignificant prostate cancers.
- End-fire and side-fire ultrasound probes, along with transrectal and transperineal approaches to prostate biopsy, have similar cancer detection rates and complications.
- Magnetic resonance imaging–guided prostate biopsy has an evolving role in both initial and repeat prostate biopsy strategies, potentially improving sampling efficiency, increasing the detection of clinically significant cancers, and reducing the detection of insignificant cancers.
- Hematuria, hematospermia, and rectal bleeding are common complications of prostate needle biopsy, but are generally self-limiting and well tolerated.
- Fluoroquinolones and cephalosporins remain the recommended prophylactic antibiotics, although the frequency of quinolone-resistant infections is increasing.

OPTIMIZING PROSTATE BIOPSY IN CLINICAL PRACTICE: CORE NUMBER AND LOCATION
Cancer Detection Rate

Optimizing prostate cancer detection rates (CDRs) in clinical practice translates into defining the ideal number and location of biopsy cores to maximize clinically significant cancer detection, minimize insignificant cancer detection, and reduce the necessity for repetitive rebiopsy. The recently published American Urological Association (AUA) recommendations on the optimal technique of prostate biopsy and specimen handling,[1] along with an accompanying review article,[2] recommended the use of an extended 12-core biopsy strategy, incorporating far-lateral and apical samples, for initial prostate biopsy. Historically, comparison of CDR between sextant biopsy protocols and extended-core biopsy protocols (involving 10–12 cores) have demonstrated a trend of increasing CDR with greater core number (**Table 1**).[3] Although increasing the cores from 6 to 12 results in a significant increase in CDR, increasing the number of cores to 18 or 21 (saturation biopsy) as an initial biopsy strategy does not appear to result in a similar increase.[4] de la Taille and colleagues[5] found in their cohort of 303 patients that the CDRs using sextant, extended 12-core, 18-core, and 21-core biopsy schemes

M.A. Bjurlin and J.S. Wysock: Supported in part by grant UL1 TR000038 from the National Center for the Advancement of Translational Science (NCATS), National Institutes of Health; All authors: Supported in part by the Joseph and Diane Steinberg Charitable Trust.
Division of Urologic Oncology, Department of Urology, New York University Langone Medical Center, 32nd Street, 2nd Floor, New York, NY 10016, USA
* Corresponding author.
E-mail address: Samir.taneja@nyumc.org

Urol Clin N Am 41 (2014) 299–313
http://dx.doi.org/10.1016/j.ucl.2014.01.011
0094-0143/14/$ – see front matter © 2014 Elsevier Inc. All rights reserved.

Table 1
Cancer detection rates by number of prostate biopsy cores

	Cancer Detection Rate				
No. of Prostate Biopsy Cores	6	10–12	18	20–21	24
Study					
Eskew et al, 1997	26.1%	40.3%[a]	—	—	—
Naughton et al, 2000	26%	27%	—	—	—
Presti et al, 2000	33.5%	39.7%	—	—	—
Babaian et al, 2000	20%	30%	—	—	—
Elabbady & Khedr, 2006	24.8%	36.4%	—	—	—
Gore et al, 2001	31%	43%	—	—	—
Philip et al, 2004	23%	32%	—	—	—
Shim et al, 2007	22%	28%	—	—	—
Scattoni et al, 2008	—	38.5%	39.9%	—	—
de la Taille et al, 2003	22.7%	28.3%	30.7%	31.3%	—
Pepe & Aragona, 2007	—	39.8%	39.8%	—	49.0%[b]
Jones et al, 2006	—	52%	—	—	45%
Guichard et al, 2007	—	38.7%	41.5%	42.5%	—
Ploussard et al, 2012	32.5%	40.4%	—	43.3%	—

[a] 13-Core extended-biopsy strategy.
[b] 29-Core saturation-biopsy strategy.
Data from Refs.[3–5,19,123–132]

were 22.7%, 28.3%, 30.7%, and 31.3%, respectively. Diagnostic yield improved by 24.7% when the number of cores increased from 6 to 12, but only by 10.6% when the number of cores increased from 12 to 21. In their review of the diagnostic value of systematic prostate biopsies, Eichler and colleagues[6] noted that taking more than 12 cores did not significantly improve cancer yield.

With regard to core location, the AUA white paper highlights the need to sample both apical and far-lateral regions as these appear to increase CDR, but notes that transition-zone sampling does not improve prostate CDR at initial extended biopsy. In a study by Babaian and colleagues[3] evaluating an 11-core biopsy strategy in 362 patients, the CDR was 34% among 85 men undergoing primary biopsy. Among 9 cancers identified uniquely at nonsextant sites, 7 were identified by anterior-horn (far-lateral) biopsies and 2 by transition-zone biopsies. Because the entire apex is composed of peripheral zone, biopsies performed at the apex or lateral apex might not sample the anterior apex. Biopsy cores directed at the anterior apex exclusively contribute to cancer detection in 4% to 6% of men.[7] Moreover, additional extreme anterior apical cores (one on each side) have achieved the highest rate of unique cancer detection ($P = .011$).[8] Transition-zone biopsies, as part of an initial diagnostic strategy,

have generally demonstrated a low rate of exclusive cancer detection (2.9%),[9] although in some series CDR did improve with transition-zone sampling ($P = .023$).[4]

Likelihood of Clinically Significant/Insignificant Prostate Cancer

Among the growing concerns of overdetection of prostate cancer, a potential drawback of increasing core numbers at the time of initial biopsy is the increased likelihood of detecting insignificant prostate cancers. Few reports have shown a higher detection rate of clinically insignificant prostate cancer with extended-biopsy schemes in comparison with sextant,[10] while most studies found no significant differences in the detection rate of insignificant cancers between sextant and extended-biopsy schemes.[11] In a large database study (N = 4072), Meng and colleagues[11] found that increasing the number of biopsy cores did not result in the identification of a disproportionate number of lower-risk tumors. However, increasing the number of cores beyond the extended-biopsy strategy does appear to increase the rate of indolent cancer detection. Haas and colleagues[12] showed that an extended-biopsy 18-core strategy increased the detection rate of insignificant prostate cancers by 22%. Far-lateral and apical-directed biopsy cores do not appear to increase the detection of insignificant cancers while the CDR of the transition-zone sample is already low.[2]

Negative Predictive Value/Avoidance of Repeat Biopsy

Sextant biopsies have false-negative rates of 15% to 34% based on CDR at the time of repeat biopsy and computer simulation.[13,14] Levine and colleagues[14] first evaluated the use of a 12-core biopsy, using 2 consecutive sets of sextant biopsy in a single sitting, and demonstrated an increase in cancer detection to 31% overall, with only 21% being detected on the first sextant alone. Other researchers have demonstrated that prostate CDRs on repeat biopsy vary as a function of the extent of the initial biopsy.[15] If a prior negative biopsy used a sextant scheme, the CDR was 39% with a repeat extended biopsy, whereas if a prior negative biopsy used an extended scheme, the CDR of the repeat biopsy decreased to 21% to 28%. Use of repeat saturation (20–24 cores) biopsy after initial saturation biopsy has been shown to have a CDR of 24%, similar to the CDR of 29% for biopsies following an initial sextant biopsy ($P = .08$).[15] These investigators concluded that the false-negative rate for repeat prostate biopsies after an initial saturation biopsy is equivalent to that following traditional biopsy, and recommended against saturation prostate biopsy for primary biopsy.

Although it has been demonstrated that T1c cancers are present in the transition zone more frequently than T2 cancers, the yield of routine transition-zone biopsy remains low.[9,16,17] Because relatively few cancers are found uniquely in the transition zone, it is unlikely that repeat biopsies would be avoided by routine transition-zone sampling. No difference has been seen in the number of men requiring a repeat biopsy when evaluating the role of transition-zone sampling on initial and repeat biopsy.[17] Sampling the anterior apical peripheral zone on repeat biopsy identified 36.0% with cancer exclusively in the anterior apical peripheral-zone cores. The CDR from the anterior apical peripheral-zone sites was significantly higher in the repeat biopsies than in the initial biopsies ($P<.01$), suggesting a predominance of missed cancers in this location.[18] Apical cores and extreme anterior apical cores have been shown to increase unique cancer detection, and to minimize the potential for misdiagnosis and the need for repeat biopsy.[8] Few studies have evaluated the negative predictive value (NPV) of far-lateral sampling of the prostate. However, lateral sampling appears to improve clinical NPV because several cancers are identified only in the lateral sample.

Pathologic Concordance Between Biopsy and Radical Prostatectomy

Several studies have demonstrated that extended-biopsy schemes improve biopsy concordance with prostatectomy specimens. Concordance rates of prostate cancer grade, when an extended-biopsy scheme is used, are as high as 85%, compared with 50% with a sextant biopsy.[19–21] Upgrading of the Gleason score has been shown to be significantly less likely with the extended scheme (17% vs 41% for the sextant scheme, $P<.001$).[20] Similarly, 14% of the prostate cancers detected using extended-biopsy schemes have been shown to be undergraded, compared with 25% of cancers detected using sextant schemes ($P = .01$).[21] The results of biopsy schemes involving saturation biopsies (>12 cores) appear to have a higher concordance rate with results from prostatectomy (59%) than a scheme involving fewer than 12 cores (47%, $P = .05$).[22]

Apical and laterally directed sampling improves the ability to predict pathologic features on prostatectomy, whereas the concordance of transition-zone biopsies with radical prostatectomy pathology is poor. In a study evaluating individually labeled, preoperative apical core biopsies and corresponding prostatectomy specimens, Rogatsch and colleagues[23] determined the positive predictive value (PPV) for identifying the tumor location correctly was 71.1%, whereas the lack of cancer in the apical biopsy had an NPV of 75.5%. Cancer concordance of transition-zone biopsies and prostatectomy specimens range from approximately 20% to 40%.[24] The role of lateral sampling of the prostate was evaluated by Singh and colleagues,[25] who showed that laterally directed cores were independent predictors of pathologic features at prostatectomy.

INFLUENCE OF BIOPSY TECHNIQUE
Transrectal

End-fire versus side-fire cancer detection rates
At present, 2 different approaches are used for transrectal prostate sampling, including an end-fire or side-fire configuration of the biopsy probe (**Fig. 1**). Evidence from retrospective studies has initially suggested that an end-fire configuration results in a greater prostate CDR than a side-fire configuration. In a study of 2674 patients, Ching and colleagues[26] evaluated 2674 patients who underwent prostate biopsy and showed a prostate CDR for end-fire versus side-fire probes of 45.8% versus 38.5%. Similar results were shown by Paul

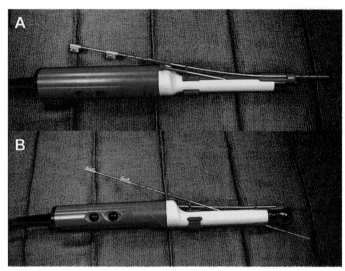

Fig. 1. End-fire (*A*) and side-fire (*B*) configurations of the transrectal ultrasound biopsy probe. (*Courtesy of Analogic Co., Peabody, MA; with permission.*)

and colleagues[27] in a study of 2625 subjects (31.3% vs 21.5%). Ching and colleagues[28] also found that the use of an end-fire probe on repeat biopsy significantly increased prostate cancer detection (odds ratio [OR] 1.59, 95% confidence interval 1.03–2.46). It has been hypothesized that improved cancer detection with the end-fire approach may be due, in part, to a better ability to sample the apex, lateral regions, and the anterior gland because of its needle angle.

Although both of the aforementioned studies included large numbers of patients, they were retrospective, and the number of cores and biopsy schemes were not standardized. To address this concern, Rom and colleagues[29] performed a prospective, randomized, multicenter study comparing prostate CDRs of end-fire and side-fire transrectal ultrasound (TRUS) probe configurations. The prostate CDR did not differ between the end-fire and side-fire probes (34.3% vs 34.4%, *P* = .972). Recently, Raber and colleagues[30] confirmed these findings in a study comparing end-fire and side-fire configurations in 1705 patients undergoing first biopsy and rebiopsy. No significant difference was found between the 2 probes in the first biopsy and rebiopsy sets (38% vs 36.5%, *P* = .55; 10.8% vs 9.3%, *P* = .7). The side-fire transrectal probe has been associated with a better patient-tolerance profile.[30,31]

Computerized templates for prostate biopsy

Computerized templates offer a biopsy strategy with reliable sampling of the same locations in the prostate each time. Available platforms typically convert 2-dimensional (2D) ultrasound data to a 3-dimensional (3D) model or image of the prostate. This technique takes into account the variability in prostate volume and shape, and allows reproducible sampling through accurate needle placement, in a known and recorded location. Furthermore, in theory such a biopsy should allow better negative accuracy through reproducible spatial sampling of all essential areas of the gland. If an initial biopsy is negative for cancer, subsequent biopsies can be arrayed in such a way as to sample different regions of the prostate, which could potentially reduce sampling error. Although such schemes do not increase cancer detection, they allow more reproducible sampling, which increases the PPV with regard to cancer location. This factor has potential value in monitoring or treatment planning.

At present, 2 computerized biopsy systems are being studied for the purpose of systematic biopsy: TargetScan and Artemis. 3D transrectal prostate mapping with TargetScan performed with an endorectal ultrasound probe has been studied in 2 series. In a retrospective multicenter review, a comparative analysis of 140 TargetScan biopsies and 23 associated prostatectomy specimens demonstrated pathologic concordance in 52%.[32] In a single-institution study, a simulation on 20 radical prostatectomy specimens showed that TargetScan biopsy correctly identified cancer in 16 (80%) of the glands. This technique was reproducible between different operators, as demonstrated by an 85% concordance of biopsy cores.[33]

Artemis is a 3D imaging and navigation system that converts 2D monochromatic ultrasound images to an enhanced 3D color image allowing manipulation, planning, and management of the prostate biopsy process (**Fig. 2**). While capable

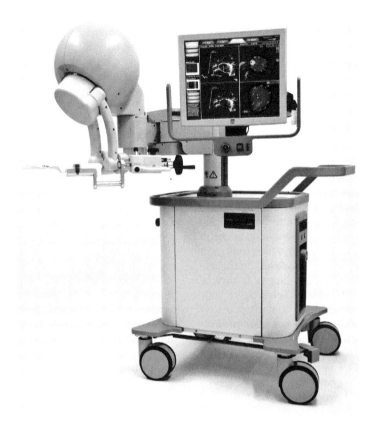

Fig. 2. Artemis 3-dimensional imaging and navigation system. (*Courtesy of* Eigen, Grass Valley, CA; with permission.)

of performing a computer-directed template biopsy, as in the case of TargetScan, Artemis is distinct in that spatial-tracking of the arm provides exact recording of the location of the biopsy core, thus allowing the user to return to the previous biopsy site at a later setting if considering surveillance or rebiopsy. Natarajan and colleagues[34] completed Artemis biopsy in 180 of 218 men. In the tracking study, they were able to return to the same needle position with a recorded error of 1.2 mm ± 1.1 mm.

Magnetic Resonance Imaging–Guided Prostate Biopsy

Whereas conventional biopsy has relied on improving sampling through increasing numbers of cores, an alternative approach is to reduce sampling error through localization. Recent improvements in multiparametric magnetic resonance imaging (MRI) have allowed accurate localization of prostate cancer.[35,36] Several investigators have evaluated the impact on cancer detection of prebiopsy MRI followed by targeted biopsy. The use of MRI-targeted biopsy has been studied in the setting of previous negative biopsy,[37] men with no

history of previous biopsy,[38] and, most recently, those on active surveillance.[39,40]

Among men undergoing repeat biopsy, 54% were found to have cancer only identified on the MRI-targeted cores. Cancers in this setting are most often found in the anterior prostate or apex.[7] Among men presenting with no previous history of cancer, prebiopsy MRI seems to have the potential to stratify the risk of prostate cancer through the application of a suspicion score.[41,42] In a study of 555 men, Haffner and colleagues[43] demonstrated that MRI-targeted biopsy identified fewer cancers overall when compared with systematic biopsy (236 of 302 vs 290 of 302), but detected a comparable number of clinically significant cancers (236 of 249 vs 237 of 249). All cancers detected by the MRI-targeted approach were deemed significant. In addition, more cancer was identified per core, suggesting the potential for more accurate risk stratification. Several subsequent studies have shown similar results[44] suggesting a potential to use MRI not only to improve cancer detection but also to reduce overdetection of indolent disease. The ability to improve risk stratification through better sampling of cancer has also been suggested by several studies evaluating the impact of MRI-targeted biopsy in active surveillance patients.[45–47]

REPEAT PROSTATE BIOPSY
Indications

High-grade intraepithelial neoplasia, atypical small acinar proliferation, and rising prostate-specific antigen

There is no consensus regarding the need for repeat biopsy in men with previous negative sampling. Potential indications include abnormal histology, rising prostate-specific antigen (PSA), or persistence of an elevated PSA. Historically, men diagnosed with isolated high-grade intraepithelial neoplasia (HGPIN) were recommended to undergo immediate repeat biopsy given the high likelihood of concordant occult cancer; however, on the implementation of extended-core biopsy in clinical practice it was noted that the likelihood of cancer detection on immediate repeat biopsy was small.[48] The recent European Association of Urology (EAU), AUA, and National Comprehensive Cancer Network (NCCN) guidelines reported that the presence of HGPIN diagnosis no longer represents an indication for immediate repeat biopsy.[49] Epstein and Herawi[50] have asserted that the risk of prostate cancer at repeat prostate biopsy after HGPIN diagnosis (22%) is similar to the risk of cancer detection after an initial benign biopsy. In addition, prospective trials have failed to demonstrate an association between the presence of HGPIN at initial prostate biopsy and subsequent prostate cancer at repeat prostate biopsy.[51,52] However, studies by Benecchi and colleagues[53] and Netto and Epstein[54] have identified the presence of HGPIN as a risk factor in their analyses, and included HGPIN in their repeat prostate biopsy nomograms.

The number of HGPIN foci appears to be an important prognosticator, and influences the suggested management protocols. For example, Godoy and colleagues[55] and Merrimen and colleagues[56] have found that isolated HGPIN does not warrant any further prostate biopsy. Similarly, data from the Cleveland Clinic have shown that on comparison of men with multifocal and isolated HGPIN on initial saturation biopsy, an 80% and 0% likelihood of prostate cancer on repeat prostate biopsy was observed, respectively.[57] Taken together, these findings demonstrate that a single focus may have limited clinical significance, with minimally increased risk of the development of prostate cancer. Multifocal HGPIN, however, more than doubles the risk of subsequent cancer detection. The NCCN guidelines recommend that for patients with multifocal HGPIN (≥2 cores) on an extended pattern biopsy, repeat biopsy be performed within the first year.

Another critical predictor of cancer risk in men with isolated HGPIN is the interval to biopsy. Studies of serial delayed interval biopsy suggest that repeat biopsy can be performed at intervals longer than 1 year.[48,55] The authors' group has advocated serial prostate biopsy every 3 years based on early observation of prostate cancer in 26% of men biopsied 3 years after initial diagnosis and subsequent demonstration of a similar persistent risk on 6-year biopsy.[48] Among a large cohort of men with isolated HGPIN followed for 3 years as part of the placebo arm of a chemoprevention trial, cancer was demonstrated in 34.7% of men with serial biopsy performed each year.[58]

The natural history of atypical small acinar proliferation (ASAP) is less well defined than that of HGPIN; however, if ASAP is present in the initial biopsy specimen, the risk of diagnosing prostate cancer on subsequent biopsy is significantly increased. Unlike HGPIN, ASAP represents uncertainty regarding the diagnosis of cancer. Studies of repeat biopsy have shown a detection rate for prostatic adenocarcinoma as high as 55% after an initial diagnosis of ASAP[59] and up to 58% when found in combination with HGPIN on initial biopsy.[60] Regardless of PSA values, current recommendations are to rebiopsy all patients with ASAP in their initial biopsy specimen within 3 to 6 months. The typical technique of biopsy is focal saturation to the region of observed atypia.

A rising PSA after a negative prostate biopsy may indicate undiagnosed cancer, and a persistently elevated PSA may draw concern of a missed occult cancer. A rising PSA after a negative prostate biopsy or a persistently elevated PSA may draw concern of a missed occult cancer. An important consideration is adequacy of the initial prostate biopsy, taking into account the number of cores taken and anatomic sites sampled, areas of undersampling, length of each core, and quality of the tissues sampled. Most studies of repeat prostate biopsy following extended initial biopsy indicate that up to 30% of patients have cancers that were not previously identified.[61,62] A repeat biopsy strategy may include focal saturation, extended 21-core biopsy, saturation biopsy, or image guidance to improve the detection rate.

Technique

Focal saturation, 12-core biopsy, saturation biopsy

When performing repeat biopsies, it is important to recognize that the region of the prostate potentially undersampled in a 12-core biopsy scheme is the anterior apex.[7] The entire apex of the prostate is composed of peripheral zone and, although extended schemes do sample the apex and lateral apex, additional cores should be taken from the anterior apex on repeat biopsy. Similarly, repeat biopsy should include the transition zone, as supported by the EAU guidelines.[63]

The precise labeling of the initial prostate locations is important to direct rebiopsy in a more concentrated fashion into the region of the initial ASAP.[50,64] Allen and colleagues[64] demonstrated earlier that the chance of detecting prostate cancer greatly increases by performing a rebiopsy not only of the atypical site but also of adjacent contralateral and adjacent ipsilateral areas. However, Scattoni and colleagues[65] has more recently reported that a precise spatial concordance between ASAP and prostate cancer was present in only 33% of the cases, similar to the likelihood of finding prostate cancer in an adjacent or a nonadjacent site.

Contemporary recommendations for the technique of repeat prostate biopsy suggests that a repeated 10-core to 12-core extended-biopsy scheme remains the most frequently used technique, with additional cores from suspected areas by modern imaging of the anterior and transition zone. In comparison with standard extended techniques (10–14 cores), repeat saturation biopsies (20–24 cores) increase the CDR (24.9% vs 32.7%, $P = .0075$).[62]

Transperineal saturation biopsy
According to AUA and NCCN guidelines, a saturation prostate biopsy may be considered in men with a prior negative biopsy and persistent suspicion of prostate cancer. The transperineal biopsy technique allows for improved sampling of the apex and anterior zones, which are common sites of cancer detection on repeat biopsy. In a series of 92 consecutive men with at least 2 negative prior transrectal biopsies, most of the tumors detected on transperineal saturation biopsy were found in the anterior zone (83.3%).[66] Transrectal and transperineal prostate saturation repeat biopsies have a similar CDR.[67]

MRI-targeted repeat prostate biopsy
MRI-targeted repeat biopsy has the potential to reduce the sampling error of the initial biopsy through localization of disease (**Fig. 3**). In a recent meta-regression study comparing cancer detection on repeat prostate biopsy, Nelson and colleagues[68] compared transperineal, ultrasound-guided transrectal saturation, and MRI-targeted biopsy whereby CDRs were 30.0%, 36.8%, and 37.6%, respectively. Meta-regression analysis showed that MRI-targeted biopsy had significantly higher cancer detection than transperineal biopsy. However, there were no significant differences between median Gleason scores among the 3 biopsy strategies. The investigators concluded that in the rebiopsy setting, it is unclear as to which strategy offers the highest CDR. However, MRI-targeted biopsies may potentially detect more prostate cancers than other modalities, and can achieve this with fewer biopsy cores.

PAIN CONTROL
Technique of Anesthesia

Improvements in anesthesia techniques have allowed urologists to sample a greater number of cores, and from different locations in the gland,

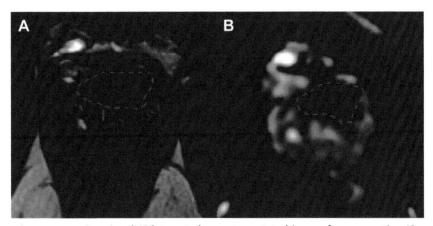

Fig. 3. Magnetic resonance imaging (MRI)-targeted repeat prostate biopsy after a negative 12-core template biopsy. MRI demonstrated a left anterior mid-to-apex transition-zone lesion that appeared to intimately involve anterior fibromuscular stroma (suspicion score 4/5) on T2-weighted imaging (A) and apparent diffusion coefficient map (B). Targeted biopsy revealed Gleason score 3 + 4 = 7 prostate cancer in 2 of 2 cores, 20% to 70% of each core.

including the ability to perform a saturation biopsy procedure in an office setting.[62] Both rectal and prostatic anesthesia may limit pain during the procedure. Intrarectal local anesthesia has been used, as lubrication to reduce friction and protect the mucosa during instrumentation as well as to ease the discomfort on introduction of the ultrasound probe. A variety of anesthetic agents have been used, including lidocaine, prilocaine, nifedipine, and dimethyl sulfoxide, in various combinations and with varied results. A periprostatic nerve block is commonly used in TRUS-guided biopsy whereby the optimal injection site seems to be localized in the angle between the prostate and the seminal vesicles, which can be easily identified as a hypoechoic area on TRUS. A concentration of 1% lidocaine, 5 mL per side, is sufficient to provide pain relief. Periprostatic nerve block is associated with significantly less pain during biopsy than is lidocaine gel or placebo,[69] and is superior to intrarectal instillation of anesthetic cream.[70] Extensive biopsy protocols may be comfortably performed in the office setting using local anesthesia with 22 mL 1% lidocaine injection.[71] Despite lack of a standardized dose or optimal technique, periprostatic anesthetic infiltration should be considered the gold standard.[72] Intraprostatic anesthesia has been provided in combination with periprostatic nerve block resulting in improved pain control,[73] but further studies are needed to delineate location, technique, and dosages. Historically the transperineal approach to prostate biopsy has been performed under general anesthesia, but recent studies have demonstrated that the combination of pudendal and periprostatic nerve block is well tolerated and improves pain reduction without the need for general anesthesia.[74]

COMPLICATIONS
Incidence of Prostate Biopsy Complications

According to the AUA clinical guidelines on the incidence, prevention, and complications related to prostate needle biopsy, the most common urologic side effects of a prostate needle biopsy include hematuria, rectal bleeding, hematospermia, urinary tract infection, and acute urinary retention.[75,76] Erectile dysfunction and vasovagal response have also been noted to occur in patients undergoing prostate biopsy (**Table 2**).

Bleeding Complications

Episodes of significant bleeding after prostate biopsy may occur in 1% to 4% of patients.[77] Recent data suggest that hematuria is noted in 23% to 84%, rectal bleeding in 17% to 45%, and

Table 2 Incidence of prostate biopsy complications	
Complication	Incidence (%)
Hematuria	23–84
Rectal bleeding	17–45
Hematospermia	12–93
Urinary tract infection	2–6
Bacteremia	0.1–2.2
Hospitalization	0.6–4.1
Erectile dysfunction	2.2
Urinary retention	1–7
Vasovagal response	1.4–5.3

Data from Refs.[5,78–80,95,96,98,112,117,118,120–122]

hematospermia in 12% to 93% of men after prostate needle biopsy. However, relatively fewer men who underwent a biopsy perceived hematuria (6%), rectal bleeding (3%), and hematospermia as a major to moderate problem (27%).[5,78–80]

Prevention of prostate biopsy complications

Current considerations for the prevention of bleeding complications after prostate biopsy include holding anticoagulation, including warfarin, aspirin, nonsteroidal anti-inflammatory drugs (NSAIDs), herbal supplements, and clopidogrel, for 7 to 10 days before the biopsy when it is possible to do so. For those patients with underlying coagulopathy or who are on warfarin, prostatic biopsy should not be performed until the international normalized ratio has been corrected to lower than 1.5. Several studies have evaluated the safety of maintaining anticoagulation during biopsy. Available data suggest that stopping aspirin may be unnecessary, as it does not increase the incidence or severity of bleeding complications.[81–83] However, aspirin may prolong the duration of self-limiting hematuria and rectal bleeding.[81,83] Similar trends demonstrating no increased risk of bleeding have been noted in evaluating the safety of continuing warfarin during biopsy.[84,85] Taken together, the data suggest that aspirin may be continued during the procedure if there is any concern about the safety of withholding it. Data on stopping warfarin and clopidogrel are limited, and the risks between cardiovascular or thromboembolic events when stopping anticoagulation must be weighed against the risk for bleeding and associated complications with continuation.[76]

Influence of technique

In a meta-analysis and review of prostate biopsy results, Shen and colleagues[86] found no significant differences in the incidence of major or minor complications between the transperineal and transrectal techniques. In prospective randomized study comparing transperineal with transrectal systematic 12-core biopsy, Hara and colleagues[87] found no differences in rectal bleeding, hematuria, or hematospermia between the two techniques. A major consideration is the potential to reduce infection by way of a transrectal approach, particularly in view of the increasing rate of infection following biopsy noted in recent years.[88]

Management

Severe rectal bleeding may be managed initially with bed rest, volume resuscitation, and transfusion. If the patient's condition does not improve while under observation, options for management include digital compression, rectal tamponade with a tampon,[89] inflated condom, or inflated Foley catheter balloon.[90] Colonoscopy with injection of epinephrine and polidocanol or use of sclerotherapeutic agents, angiography with embolization,[91] transrectal exploration, and suturing are alternative means of stopping rectal bleeding.[92,93] Hematuria may be managed similarly with bed rest, volume resuscitation, and transfusion. Cystoscopy or anoscopy with coagulation of bleeding points may be used in more severe cases.

Infectious Complications

Most infectious complications after prostate biopsy are limited to symptomatic urinary tract infection and low-grade febrile illness, which can be readily treated with oral or intravenous antibiotics; however, postbiopsy sepsis has emerged as a risk for this procedure. The incidence of infectious complications following prostate biopsy in large multi-institutional studies ranges from 0.1% to 7%, depending on the antimicrobial prophylactic regimen used,[88,94,95] with approximately 30% to 50% of these patients having accompanying bacteremia.[96,97] The risk of hospitalization for infectious complications in contemporary studies ranges from 0.6% to 4.1%.[95] The reported incidence of urinary tract infection after prostate biopsy typically ranges between 2% and 6%.[98] Bacteremia is frequently accompanied by severe sepsis, which has an overall incidence of 0.1% to 2.2% following prostate biopsy.[96] One recent study reported that among post–TRUS biopsy patients hospitalized with *Escherichia coli* bacteremia, 25% had severe sepsis requiring admission to the intensive care unit.[99] In terms of repeat prostate biopsy, Loeb and colleagues[100] demonstrated that a repeat biopsy session was not associated with a greater risk of infectious (OR 0.81, P = .39) or serious noninfectious urologic complications (OR 0.94, P = .82) in comparison with the initial biopsy.

Prevention

According to the AUA Best Practice Statement, TRUS-guided prostate biopsy, performed through a grossly contaminated field, requires important preventive considerations. There is wide variation in the approach to the preparation of the rectum. Some studies found no benefit to either preprocedural povidone-iodine[96] or sodium biphosphate enemas.[101] However, another study found that a bisacodyl suppository rectal preparation the night before or on the morning of the procedure decreased infectious complications.[102]

The AUA Best Practice Policy Statement on Urologic Surgery Antimicrobial Prophylaxis recommends a fluoroquinolone or first-/second-/third-generation cephalosporin before biopsy.[103] At present, no conclusive data have been found to support the use of long-course (3 days) over short-course (1 day) fluoroquinolone regimens, or multiple-dose versus single-dose schedules.[104] Although antibiotic prophylaxis is largely effective in preventing infection, leading to a low incidence of sepsis, recently there have been an increase in the incidence of quinolone-resistant infection resulting from more frequent use of quinolones in the population overall, including at the time of transrectal prostate biopsy.[105] Prebiopsy screening with rectal swabs may allow identification of those men harboring antibiotic resistant organisms in their endogenous gastrointestinal flora prebiopsy, and for whom fluoroquinolone prophylaxis may not be appropriate.[94] This strategy has revealed a prevalence of about 22% of men harboring fluoroquinolone-resistant bacteria.[94,106] Taylor and colleagues[107] targeted specific antimicrobial prophylaxis based on rectal swab results. These investigators were able to show a nonsignificant reduction in post–prostate biopsy infections from 2.6% to 0% (P = .12) and a potential cost saving per infectious complication averted. However, these methods have not been broadly used, and the determination of true benefit requires further prospective investigation.

The need for routine urine culture before prostate biopsy is unclear; urine culture seems only to be useful in the decision to refrain from prostate biopsy when bacterial growth is evident.[108] The use of urinalysis or urine dipstick before prostate biopsy is widespread, even though there are no published studies to document its benefit.

Technique

In a prospective randomized study comparing transperineal and transrectal systematic 12-core prostate biopsy, Hara and colleagues[87] found no differences in the rates sepsis or postbiopsy fevers. Similarly, Miller and colleagues[109] found similar rates of sepsis when comparing the two biopsy techniques. Shen and colleagues[86] determined that there was no significant difference in the incidence of major or minor complications between the transperineal and transrectal techniques in a large meta-analysis.

Management

At present, there are no published guidelines for the management of post–prostate biopsy infections. However, in addition to patient-specific prophylactic regimens, consideration should be given to empiric followed by culture-driven antimicrobial therapy if a patient presents with postbiopsy sepsis. Previous studies have demonstrated that inappropriate empiric therapy for E coli bloodstream infections is associated with an increased risk of mortality.[110] Broader-spectrum empiric antimicrobial coverage should be considered for post–prostate biopsy sepsis against that given for other causes of community-onset urosepsis, as prostate biopsy was actually a risk factor for bacteremia with multidrug-resistant E coli.[99] Other individual risk factors that should be considered when choosing appropriate empiric therapy include prior exposure to fluoroquinolones. Initial therapy must cover E coli, the most common pathogen, as well as numerous other organisms. Before treatment a urine culture, and blood cultures if the patient is febrile, should be obtained.

Quality of Life

Erectile dysfunction

Recent data have suggested an association between prostate biopsy, lower urinary tract symptoms, and erectile dysfunction. In their randomized trial of 145 men, Klein and colleagues[111] found that prostate biopsy may cause urinary symptoms and erectile dysfunction regardless of anesthesia or number of cores sampled, as shown by a decrease in IIEF-5 (International Index of Erectile Dysfunction) and an increase in IPSS (International Prostate Symptom Score) in their study. Erectile dysfunction was noted in 2.2% of men in a study be Akyol and Adayener,[112] possibly attributable to nerve injury caused by the biopsy needle. However, in a study by Helfand and colleagues,[113] cancer diagnosis appears to have an adverse effect on the erectile function of men undergoing prostate biopsy but no effect on lower urinary tract symptoms. Similarly, serial prostate biopsies appear to have an adverse effect on erectile function in men with prostate cancer on active surveillance, but do not affect lower urinary tract symptoms.[114] Several other studies, however, have suggested the effects of

the prostate needle biopsy are transient, with no significant differences in men with and without prostate cancer.[115,116]

Urinary retention

Urinary retention requiring temporary catheterization develops in up to 1% of men undergoing transrectal prostate biopsy.[80,117,118] Men with enlarged glands and higher IPSS are more prone to develop postbiopsy retention.[118] Data suggest that starting higher-risk patients on an α-blocker before prostate biopsy may prevent episodes of urinary retention.[119] Higher rates of acute urinary retention have been noted in men undergoing transperineal prostate biopsy.[120]

Other

Excessive anxiety and discomfort from the endorectal probe may produce a moderate or severe vasovagal response in 1.4% to 5.3% of patients[121,122] and may require termination of the procedure. Placing the patient in the Trendelenburg position and use of intravenous hydration usually resolve these symptoms, with further intervention as clinically indicated.

SUMMARY

A 12-core systematic biopsy that incorporates apical and far-lateral cores in the template distribution allows maximal cancer detection and avoidance of a repeat biopsy, while minimizing the detection of insignificant prostate cancers. MRI-targeted prostate biopsy has an evolving role in both initial and repeat prostate biopsy strategies, potentially improving sampling efficiency, increasing the detection of clinically significant cancers, and reducing the detection of insignificant cancers. Hematuria, hematospermia, and rectal bleeding are common complications of prostate needle biopsy, but are generally self-limiting and well tolerated. All men should receive antimicrobial prophylaxis before biopsy. Fluoroquinolones or cephalosporins remain the recommended prophylactic antibiotics, although the frequency of quinolone-resistant infections is increasing.

REFERENCES

1. Taneja SS, Bjurlin MA, Carter HB, et al. White paper: AUA/Optimal techniques of prostate biopsy and specimen handling. 2013. Available at: http://www.auanet.org/common/pdf/education/clinical-guidance/Prostate-Biopsy-WhitePaper.pdf. Accessed May 15, 2013.
2. Bjurlin MA, Carter HB, Schellhammer P, et al. Optimization of initial prostate biopsy in clinical

practice: sampling, labeling and specimen processing. J Urol 2013;189:2039–46.

3. Babaian RJ, Toi A, Kamoi K, et al. A comparative analysis of sextant and an extended 11-core multisite directed biopsy strategy. J Urol 2000;163:152–7.

4. Guichard G, Larre S, Gallina A, et al. Extended 21-sample needle biopsy protocol for diagnosis of prostate cancer in 1000 consecutive patients. Eur Urol 2007;52:430–5.

5. de la Taille A, Antiphon P, Salomon L, et al. Prospective evaluation of a 21-sample needle biopsy procedure designed to improve the prostate cancer detection rate. Urology 2003;61:1181–6.

6. Eichler K, Hempel S, Wilby J, et al. Diagnostic value of systematic biopsy methods in the investigation of prostate cancer: a systematic review. J Urol 2006;175:1605–12.

7. Meng MV, Franks JH, Presti JC Jr, et al. The utility of apical anterior horn biopsies in prostate cancer detection. Urol Oncol 2003;21:361–5.

8. Moussa AS, Meshref A, Schoenfield L, et al. Importance of additional "extreme" anterior apical needle biopsies in the initial detection of prostate cancer. Urology 2010;75:1034–9.

9. Bazinet M, Karakiewicz PI, Aprikian AG, et al. Value of systematic transition zone biopsies in the early detection of prostate cancer. J Urol 1996;155:605–6.

10. Singh H, Canto EI, Shariat SF, et al. Improved detection of clinically significant, curable prostate cancer with systematic 12-core biopsy. J Urol 2004;171:1089–92.

11. Meng MV, Elkin EP, DuChane J, et al. Impact of increased number of biopsies on the nature of prostate cancer identified. J Urol 2006;176:63–8.

12. Haas GP, Delongchamps NB, Jones RF, et al. Needle biopsies on autopsy prostates: sensitivity of cancer detection based on true prevalence. J Natl Cancer Inst 2007;99:1484–9.

13. Chen ME, Troncoso P, Johnston DA, et al. Optimization of prostate biopsy strategy using computer based analysis. J Urol 1997;158:2168–75.

14. Levine MA, Ittman M, Melamed J, et al. Two consecutive sets of transrectal ultrasound guided sextant biopsies of the prostate for the detection of prostate cancer. J Urol 1998;159:471–5.

15. Lane BR, Zippe CD, Abouassaly R, et al. Saturation technique does not decrease cancer detection during followup after initial prostate biopsy. J Urol 2008;179:1746–50.

16. Fleshner NE, Fair WR. Indications for transition zone biopsy in the detection of prostatic carcinoma. J Urol 1997;157:556–8.

17. Terris MK, Pham TQ, Issa MM, et al. Routine transition zone and seminal vesicle biopsies in all patients undergoing transrectal ultrasound guided prostate biopsies are not indicated. J Urol 1997;157:204–6.

18. Orikasa K, Ito A, Ishidoya S, et al. Anterior apical biopsy: is it useful for prostate cancer detection? Int J Urol 2008;15:900–4.

19. Elabbady AA, Khedr MM. Extended 12-core prostate biopsy increases both the detection of prostate cancer and the accuracy of Gleason score. Eur Urol 2006;49:49–53.

20. Mian BM, Lehr DJ, Moore CK, et al. Role of prostate biopsy schemes in accurate prediction of Gleason scores. Urology 2006;67:379–83.

21. San Francisco IF, DeWolf WC, Rosen S, et al. Extended prostate needle biopsy improves concordance of Gleason grading between prostate needle biopsy and radical prostatectomy. J Urol 2003;169:136–40.

22. Kahl P, Wolf S, Adam A, et al. Saturation biopsy improves preoperative Gleason scoring of prostate cancer. Pathol Res Pract 2009;205:259–64.

23. Rogatsch H, Horninger W, Volgger H, et al. Radical prostatectomy: the value of preoperative, individually labeled apical biopsies. J Urol 2000;164:754–7.

24. Haarer CF, Gopalan A, Tickoo SK, et al. Prostatic transition zone directed needle biopsies uncommonly sample clinically relevant transition zone tumors. J Urol 2009;182:1337–41.

25. Singh H, Canto EI, Shariat SF, et al. Six additional systematic lateral cores enhance sextant biopsy prediction of pathological features at radical prostatectomy. J Urol 2004;171:204–9.

26. Ching CB, Moussa AS, Li J, et al. Does transrectal ultrasound probe configuration really matter? End fire versus side fire probe prostate cancer detection rates. J Urol 2009;181:2077–82 [discussion: 2082–3].

27. Paul R, Korzinek C, Necknig U, et al. Influence of transrectal ultrasound probe on prostate cancer detection in transrectal ultrasound-guided sextant biopsy of prostate. Urology 2004;64:532–6.

28. Ching CB, Zaytoun O, Moussa AS, et al. Type of transrectal ultrasonography probe influences prostate cancer detection rates on repeat prostate biopsy. BJU Int 2012;110:E46–9.

29. Rom M, Pycha A, Wiunig C, et al. Prospective randomized multicenter study comparing prostate cancer detection rates of end-fire and side-fire transrectal ultrasound probe configuration. Urology 2012;80:15–8.

30. Raber M, Scattoni V, Gallina A, et al. Does the transrectal ultrasound probe influence prostate cancer detection in patients undergoing an extended prostate biopsy scheme? Results of a large retrospective study. BJU Int 2012;109:672–7.

31. Moussa AS, El-Shafei A, Diaz E, et al. Identification of the variables associated with pain during transrectal ultrasonography-guided prostate biopsy in the era of periprostatic nerve block: the role of

transrectal probe configuration. BJU Int 2013; 111(8):1281–6.

32. Megwalu II, Ferguson GG, Wei JT, et al. Evaluation of a novel precision template-guided biopsy system for detecting prostate cancer. BJU Int 2008; 102:546–50.

33. Andriole GL, Bullock TL, Belani JS, et al. Is there a better way to biopsy the prostate? Prospects for a novel transrectal systematic biopsy approach. Urology 2007;70:22–6.

34. Natarajan S, Marks LS, Margolis DJ, et al. Clinical application of a 3D ultrasound-guided prostate biopsy system. Urol Oncol 2011;29:334–42.

35. Isebaert S, Van den Bergh L, Haustermans K, et al. Multiparametric MRI for prostate cancer localization in correlation to whole-mount histopathology. J Magn Reson Imaging 2013;37:1392–401.

36. Delongchamps NB, Rouanne M, Flam T, et al. Multiparametric magnetic resonance imaging for the detection and localization of prostate cancer: combination of T2-weighted, dynamic contrast-enhanced and diffusion-weighted imaging. BJU Int 2011;107:1411–8.

37. Sonn GA, Chang E, Natarajan S, et al. Value of targeted prostate biopsy using magnetic resonance-ultrasound fusion in men with prior negative biopsy and elevated prostate-specific antigen. Eur Urol 2013. [Epub ahead of print].

38. Park BK, Park JW, Park SY, et al. Prospective evaluation of 3-T MRI performed before initial transrectal ultrasound-guided prostate biopsy in patients with high prostate-specific antigen and no previous biopsy. AJR Am J Roentgenol 2011;197: W876–81.

39. Vargas HA, Akin O, Afaq A, et al. Magnetic resonance imaging for predicting prostate biopsy findings in patients considered for active surveillance of clinically low risk prostate cancer. J Urol 2012; 188:1732–8.

40. Margel D, Yap SA, Lawrentschuk N, et al. Impact of multiparametric endorectal coil prostate magnetic resonance imaging on disease reclassification among active surveillance candidates: a prospective cohort study. J Urol 2012;187:1247–52.

41. Barentsz JO, Richenberg J, Clements R, et al. ESUR prostate MR guidelines 2012. Eur Radiol 2012;22:746–57.

42. Rosenkrantz AB, Kim S, Lim RP, et al. Prostate cancer localization using multiparametric MR imaging: comparison of Prostate Imaging Reporting and Data System (PI-RADS) and Likert Scales. Radiology 2013;269(2):482–92.

43. Haffner J, Lemaitre L, Puech P, et al. Role of magnetic resonance imaging before initial biopsy: comparison of magnetic resonance imaging-targeted and systematic biopsy for significant prostate cancer detection. BJU Int 2011;108:E171–8.

44. Marks L, Young S, Natarajan S. MRI-ultrasound fusion for guidance of targeted prostate biopsy. Curr Opin Urol 2013;23:43–50.

45. Park BH, Jeon HG, Choo SH, et al. Role of multiparametric 3.0 tesla magnetic resonance imaging in prostate cancer patients eligible for active surveillance. BJU Int 2013. [Epub ahead of print].

46. Stamatakis L, Siddiqui MM, Nix JW, et al. Accuracy of multiparametric magnetic resonance imaging in confirming eligibility for active surveillance for men with prostate cancer. Cancer 2013;119: 3359–66.

47. Mullins JK, Bonekamp D, Landis P, et al. Multiparametric magnetic resonance imaging findings in men with low-risk prostate cancer followed using active surveillance. BJU Int 2013;111:1037–45.

48. Lefkowitz GK, Taneja SS, Brown J, et al. Followup interval prostate biopsy 3 years after diagnosis of high grade prostatic intraepithelial neoplasia is associated with high likelihood of prostate cancer, independent of change in prostate specific antigen levels. J Urol 2002;168:1415–8.

49. Heidenreich A, Aus G, Bolla M, et al. EAU guidelines on prostate cancer. Eur Urol 2008;53:68–80.

50. Epstein JI, Herawi M. Prostate needle biopsies containing prostatic intraepithelial neoplasia or atypical foci suspicious for carcinoma: implications for patient care. J Urol 2006;175:820–34.

51. Gallo F, Chiono L, Gastaldi E, et al. Prognostic significance of high-grade prostatic intraepithelial neoplasia (HGPIN): risk of prostatic cancer on repeat biopsies. Urology 2008;72:628–32.

52. Gokden N, Roehl KA, Catalona WJ, et al. High-grade prostatic intraepithelial neoplasia in needle biopsy as risk factor for detection of adenocarcinoma: current level of risk in screening population. Urology 2005;65:538–42.

53. Benecchi L, Pieri AM, Melissari M, et al. A novel nomogram to predict the probability of prostate cancer on repeat biopsy. J Urol 2008;180:146–9.

54. Netto GJ, Epstein JI. Widespread high-grade prostatic intraepithelial neoplasia on prostatic needle biopsy: a significant likelihood of subsequently diagnosed adenocarcinoma. Am J Surg Pathol 2006;30:1184–8.

55. Godoy G, Huang GJ, Patel T, et al. Long-term follow-up of men with isolated high-grade prostatic intra-epithelial neoplasia followed by serial delayed interval biopsy. Urology 2011;77:669–74.

56. Merrimen JL, Jones G, Srigley JR. Is high grade prostatic intraepithelial neoplasia still a risk factor for adenocarcinoma in the era of extended biopsy sampling? Pathology 2010;42:325–9.

57. Lee MC, Moussa AS, Yu C, et al. Multifocal high grade prostatic intraepithelial neoplasia is a risk factor for subsequent prostate cancer. J Urol 2010;184:1958–62.

58. Taneja SS, Morton R, Barnette G, et al. Prostate cancer diagnosis among men with isolated high-grade intraepithelial neoplasia enrolled onto a 3-year prospective phase III clinical trial of oral toremifene. J Clin Oncol 2013;31:523–9.

59. Mancuso PA, Chabert C, Chin P, et al. Prostate cancer detection in men with an initial diagnosis of atypical small acinar proliferation. BJU Int 2007;99:49–52.

60. Scattoni V, Roscigno M, Freschi M, et al. Predictors of prostate cancer after initial diagnosis of atypical small acinar proliferation at 10 to 12 core biopsies. Urology 2005;66:1043–7.

61. Campos-Fernandes JL, Bastien L, Nicolaiew N, et al. Prostate cancer detection rate in patients with repeated extended 21-sample needle biopsy. Eur Urol 2009;55:600–6.

62. Zaytoun OM, Moussa AS, Gao T, et al. Office based transrectal saturation biopsy improves prostate cancer detection compared to extended biopsy in the repeat biopsy population. J Urol 2011;186:850–4.

63. Chun FK, Epstein JI, Ficarra V, et al. Optimizing performance and interpretation of prostate biopsy: a critical analysis of the literature. Eur Urol 2010;58:851–64.

64. Allen EA, Kahane H, Epstein JI. Repeat biopsy strategies for men with atypical diagnoses on initial prostate needle biopsy. Urology 1998;52:803–7.

65. Scattoni V, Raber M, Abdollah F, et al. Biopsy schemes with the fewest cores for detecting 95% of the prostate cancers detected by a 24-core biopsy. Eur Urol 2010;57:1–8.

66. Mabjeesh NJ, Lidawi G, Chen J, et al. High detection rate of significant prostate tumours in anterior zones using transperineal ultrasound-guided template saturation biopsy. BJU Int 2012;110:993–7.

67. Abdollah F, Novara G, Briganti A, et al. Trans-rectal versus trans-perineal saturation rebiopsy of the prostate: is there a difference in cancer detection rate? Urology 2011;77:921–5.

68. Nelson AW, Harvey RC, Parker RA, et al. Repeat prostate biopsy strategies after initial negative biopsy: meta-regression comparing cancer detection of transperineal, transrectal saturation and MRI guided biopsy. PLoS One 2013;8:e57480.

69. Lynn NN, Collins GN, Brown SC, et al. Periprostatic nerve block gives better analgesia for prostatic biopsy. BJU Int 2002;90:424–6.

70. Adamakis I, Mitropoulos D, Haritopoulos K, et al. Pain during transrectal ultrasonography guided prostate biopsy: a randomized prospective trial comparing periprostatic infiltration with lidocaine with the intra-rectal instillation of lidocaine-prilocaine cream. World J Urol 2004;22:281–4.

71. Matlaga BR, Lovato JF, Hall MC. Randomized prospective trial of a novel local anesthetic technique for extensive prostate biopsy. Urology 2003;61:972–6.

72. Autorino R, De Sio M, Di Lorenzo G, et al. How to decrease pain during transrectal ultrasound guided prostate biopsy: a look at the literature. J Urol 2005;174:2091–7.

73. Cam K, Sener M, Kayikci A, et al. Combined periprostatic and intraprostatic local anesthesia for prostate biopsy: a double-blind, placebo controlled, randomized trial. J Urol 2008;180:141–4 [discussion: 144–5].

74. Iremashvili VV, Chepurov AK, Kobaladze KM, et al. Periprostatic local anesthesia with pudendal block for transperineal ultrasound-guided prostate biopsy: a randomized trial. Urology 2010;75:1023–7.

75. American Urological Association. AUA/SUNA white paper on the incidence, prevention and treatment of complications related to prostate needle biopsy. Available at: http://www.auanet.org/common/pdf/education/clinical-guidance/AUA-SUNA-PNB-White-Paper.pdf. Accessed May 21, 2013.

76. Loeb S, Vellekoop A, Ahmed HU, et al. Systematic review of complications of prostate biopsy. Eur Urol 2013;64:876–92.

77. American Urological Association. Best practice policy statement on urologic surgery antimicrobial prophylaxis. 2008. Available at: http://www.auanet.org/content/media/antimicroprop08.pdf. Accessed May 27, 2013.

78. Rosario DJ, Lane JA, Metcalfe C, et al. Short term outcomes of prostate biopsy in men tested for cancer by prostate specific antigen: prospective evaluation within ProtecT study. BMJ 2012;344:d7894.

79. Ghani KR, Dundas D, Patel U. Bleeding after transrectal ultrasonography-guided prostate biopsy: a study of 7-day morbidity after a six-, eight- and 12-core biopsy protocol. BJU Int 2004;94:1014–20.

80. Raaijmakers R, Kirkels WJ, Roobol MJ, et al. Complication rates and risk factors of 5802 transrectal ultrasound-guided sextant biopsies of the prostate within a population-based screening program. Urology 2002;60:826–30.

81. Giannarini G, Mogorovich A, Valent F, et al. Continuing or discontinuing low-dose aspirin before transrectal prostate biopsy: results of a prospective randomized trial. Urology 2007;70:501–5.

82. Maan Z, Cutting CW, Patel U, et al. Morbidity of transrectal ultrasonography-guided prostate biopsies in patients after the continued use of low-dose aspirin. BJU Int 2003;91:798–800.

83. Halliwell OT, Yadegafar G, Lane C, et al. Transrectal ultrasound-guided biopsy of the prostate: aspirin increases the incidence of minor bleeding complications. Clin Radiol 2008;63:557–61.

84. Chowdhury R, Abbas A, Idriz S, et al. Should warfarin or aspirin be stopped prior to prostate

biopsy? An analysis of bleeding complications related to increasing sample number regimes. Clin Radiol 2012;67:e64–70.

85. Ihezue CU, Smart J, Dewbury KC, et al. Biopsy of the prostate guided by transrectal ultrasound: relation between warfarin use and incidence of bleeding complications. Clin Radiol 2005;60: 459–63 [discussion: 457–8].

86. Shen PF, Zhu YC, Wei WR, et al. The results of transperineal versus transrectal prostate biopsy: a systematic review and meta-analysis. Asian J Androl 2012;14:310–5.

87. Hara R, Jo Y, Fujii T, et al. Optimal approach for prostate cancer detection as initial biopsy: prospective randomized study comparing transperineal versus transrectal systematic 12-core biopsy. Urology 2008;71:191–5.

88. Loeb S, Carter HB, Berndt SI, et al. Complications after prostate biopsy: data from SEER-Medicare. J Urol 2011;186:1830–4.

89. Maatman TJ, Bigham D, Stirling B. Simplified management of post-prostate biopsy rectal bleeding. Urology 2002;60:508.

90. Dunn IB, Underwood MJ, Kirk D. Profuse rectal bleeding after prostatic biopsy: a life-threatening complication dealt with simply. BJU Int 2000;86:910.

91. Smith JC Jr, Kerr WS, Athanasoulis CA, et al. Angiographic management of bleeding secondary to genitourinary tract surgery. J Urol 1975;113:89–92.

92. Gonen M, Resim S. Simplified treatment of massive rectal bleeding following prostate needle biopsy. Int J Urol 2004;11:570–2.

93. Pacios E, Esteban JM, Breton ML, et al. Endoscopic treatment of massive rectal bleeding following transrectal ultrasound-guided prostate biopsy. Scand J Urol Nephrol 2007;41:561–2.

94. Liss MA, Chang A, Santos R, et al. Prevalence and significance of fluoroquinolone resistant Escherichia coli in patients undergoing transrectal ultrasound guided prostate needle biopsy. J Urol 2011;185:1283–8.

95. Nam RK, Saskin R, Lee Y, et al. Increasing hospital admission rates for urological complications after transrectal ultrasound guided prostate biopsy. J Urol 2010;183:963–8.

96. Otrock ZK, Oghlakian GO, Salamoun MM, et al. Incidence of urinary tract infection following transrectal ultrasound guided prostate biopsy at a tertiary-care medical center in Lebanon. Infect Control Hosp Epidemiol 2004;25:873–7.

97. Zaytoun OM, Vargo EH, Rajan R, et al. Emergence of fluoroquinolone-resistant Escherichia coli as cause of postprostate biopsy infection: implications for prophylaxis and treatment. Urology 2011;77:1035–41.

98. Williamson DA, Barrett LK, Rogers BA, et al. Infectious complications following transrectal-ultrasound (TRUS) guided prostate biopsy: new challenges in the era of multi-drug resistant Escherichia coli. Clin Infect Dis 2013;57(2):267–74.

99. Williamson DA, Roberts SA, Paterson DL, et al. Escherichia coli bloodstream infection after transrectal ultrasound-guided prostate biopsy: implications of fluoroquinolone-resistant sequence type 131 as a major causative pathogen. Clin Infect Dis 2012;54:1406–12.

100. Loeb S, Carter HB, Berndt SI, et al. Is repeat prostate biopsy associated with a greater risk of hospitalization? Data from SEER-Medicare. J Urol 2013; 189:867–70.

101. Carey JM, Korman HJ. Transrectal ultrasound guided biopsy of the prostate. Do enemas decrease clinically significant complications? J Urol 2001;166: 82–5.

102. Jeon SS, Woo SH, Hyun JH, et al. Bisacodyl rectal preparation can decrease infectious complications of transrectal ultrasound-guided prostate biopsy. Urology 2003;62:461–6.

103. American Urological Association. Best practice policy statement on urologic surgery antimicrobial prophylaxis. 2012. Available at: http://www.auanet. org/content/media/antimicroprop08.pdf. Accessed June 2, 2013.

104. Zani EL, Clark OA, Rodrigues Netto N Jr. Antibiotic prophylaxis for transrectal prostate biopsy. Cochrane Database Syst Rev 2011;(5):CD006576.

105. Carignan A, Roussy JF, Lapointe V, et al. Increasing risk of infectious complications after transrectal ultrasound-guided prostate biopsies: time to reassess antimicrobial prophylaxis? Eur Urol 2012;62: 453–9.

106. Steensels D, Slabbaert K, De Wever L, et al. Fluoroquinolone-resistant E. coli in intestinal flora of patients undergoing transrectal ultrasound-guided prostate biopsy—should we reassess our practices for antibiotic prophylaxis? Clin Microbiol Infect 2012;18:575–81.

107. Taylor AK, Zembower TR, Nadler RB, et al. Targeted antimicrobial prophylaxis using rectal swab cultures in men undergoing transrectal ultrasound guided prostate biopsy is associated with reduced incidence of postoperative infectious complications and cost of care. J Urol 2012;187:1275–9.

108. Horcajada JP, Busto M, Grau S, et al. High prevalence of extended-spectrum beta-lactamase-producing enterobacteriaceae in bacteremia after transrectal ultrasound-guided prostate biopsy: a need for changing preventive protocol. Urology 2009;74:1195–9.

109. Miller J, Perumalla C, Heap G. Complications of transrectal versus transperineal prostate biopsy. ANZ J Surg 2005;75:48–50.

110. Tumbarello M, Trecarichi EM, Bassetti M, et al. Identifying patients harboring extended-spectrum-beta-lactamase-producing Enterobacteriaceae on

hospital admission: derivation and validation of a scoring system. Antimicrob Agents Chemother 2011;55:3485–90.

111. Klein T, Palisaar RJ, Holz A, et al. The impact of prostate biopsy and periprostatic nerve block on erectile and voiding function: a prospective study. J Urol 2010;184:1447–52.

112. Akyol I, Adayener C. Transient impotence after transrectal ultrasound-guided prostate biopsy. J Clin Ultrasound 2008;36:33–4.

113. Helfand BT, Glaser AP, Rimar K, et al. Prostate cancer diagnosis is associated with an increased risk of erectile dysfunction after prostate biopsy. BJU Int 2013;111:38–43.

114. Fujita K, Landis P, McNeil BK, et al. Serial prostate biopsies are associated with an increased risk of erectile dysfunction in men with prostate cancer on active surveillance. J Urol 2009;182:2664–9.

115. Akbal C, Turker P, Tavukcu HH, et al. Erectile function in prostate cancer-free patients who underwent prostate saturation biopsy. Eur Urol 2008;53:540–4.

116. Chrisofos M, Papatsoris AG, Dellis A, et al. Can prostate biopsies affect erectile function? Andrologia 2006;38:79–83.

117. Berger AP, Gozzi C, Steiner H, et al. Complication rate of transrectal ultrasound guided prostate biopsy: a comparison among 3 protocols with 6, 10 and 15 cores. J Urol 2004;171:1478–80 [discussion: 1480–1].

118. Zaytoun OM, Anil T, Moussa AS, et al. Morbidity of prostate biopsy after simplified versus complex preparation protocols: assessment of risk factors. Urology 2011;77:910–4.

119. Challacombe B, Dasgupta P, Patel U, et al. Recognizing and managing the complications of prostate biopsy. BJU Int 2011;108:1233–4.

120. Pepe P, Aragona F. Morbidity after transperineal prostate biopsy in 3000 patients undergoing 12 vs 18 vs more than 24 needle cores. Urology 2013;81:1142–6.

121. Djavan B, Waldert M, Zlotta A, et al. Safety and morbidity of first and repeat transrectal ultrasound guided prostate needle biopsies: results of a prospective European prostate cancer detection study. J Urol 2001;166:856–60.

122. Rodriguez LV, Terris MK. Risks and complications of transrectal ultrasound guided prostate needle biopsy: a prospective study and review of the literature. J Urol 1998;160:2115–20.

123. Eskew LA, Bare RL, McCullough DL. Systematic 5 region prostate biopsy is superior to sextant method for diagnosing carcinoma of the prostate. J Urol 1997;157:199–202 [discussion: 202–3].

124. Naughton CK, Miller DC, Mager DE, et al. A prospective randomized trial comparing 6 versus 12 prostate biopsy cores: impact on cancer detection. J Urol 2000;164:388–92.

125. Presti JC Jr, Chang JJ, Bhargava V, et al. The optimal systematic prostate biopsy scheme should include 8 rather than 6 biopsies: results of a prospective clinical trial. J Urol 2000;163:163–6.

126. Gore JL, Shariat SF, Miles BJ, et al. Optimal combinations of systematic sextant and laterally directed biopsies for the detection of prostate cancer. J Urol 2001;165:1554–9.

127. Philip J, Ragavan N, Desouza J, et al. Effect of peripheral biopsies in maximising early prostate cancer detection in 8-, 10- or 12-core biopsy regimens. BJU Int 2004;93:1218–20.

128. Shim HB, Park HK, Lee SE, et al. Optimal site and number of biopsy cores according to prostate volume prostate cancer detection in Korea. Urology 2007;69:902–6.

129. Scattoni V, Roscigno M, Raber M, et al. Initial extended transrectal prostate biopsy–are more prostate cancers detected with 18 cores than with 12 cores? J Urol 2008;179:1327–31.

130. Pepe P, Aragona F. Saturation prostate needle biopsy and prostate cancer detection at initial and repeat evaluation. Urology 2007;70:1131–5.

131. Jones JS, Patel A, Schoenfield L, et al. Saturation technique does not improve cancer detection as an initial prostate biopsy strategy. J Urol 2006;175:485–8.

132. Ploussard G, Nicolaiew N, Marchand C, et al. Prospective evaluation of an extended 21-core biopsy scheme as initial prostate cancer diagnostic strategy. Eur Urol 2012;65(1):154–61.

Screening and Detection Advances in Magnetic Resonance Image–Guided Prostate Biopsy

Samuel K. Stephenson, MS, Edward K. Chang, BS,
Leonard S. Marks, MD*

KEYWORDS

- Prostate cancer • Magnetic resonance imaging • Fusion biopsy • Targeted prostate biopsy
- Prostate-specific antigen • Ultrasonography • Transrectal ultrasonography

KEY POINTS

- Reliable imaging of prostate cancer within the organ has been elusive; however, over the past few years, use of multiparametric magnetic resonance imaging (MRI) has begun to allow visualization of many organ-confined prostate cancers. The new imaging modality and its offshoot, targeted biopsy, offer the promise of a major transformation in management of this disease.
- By aiming a biopsy needle at MRI regions of interest, a physician can now obtain tissue directly from suspicious lesions (ie, targeted prostate biopsy), rather than by blindly sampling the organ.
- Use of MRI images to guide prostate biopsy is accomplished by image fusion and may be performed in 1 of 3 ways: by direct in-bore MRI-MRI fusion; by cognitive fusion, using ultrasonography (US) guidance to sample suspicious areas on MRI; and by MRI-US fusion, using a device made for the purpose.
- MRI-US fusion devices, such as the Artemis (Eigen-Hitachi, Grass Valley, CA) or UroNav (Invivo-Philips, Gainesville, FL), allow the urologist to use sophisticated MRI images to guide prostate biopsy in an outpatient clinic setting; the procedure is contextually similar to that performed by most urologists for the past several decades.
- Targeted prostate biopsy, via MRI-US fusion, (1) allows diagnosis of serious tumors not found with conventional biopsy; (2) helps to avoid detection of insignificant tumors; (3) provides a method for repeat biopsy of specific tumor-bearing sites for men in active surveillance; and (4) creates an opportunity for study of focal therapy.

Disclosures: The project described was supported by Award Number R01CA158627 from the National Cancer Institute. The content is solely the responsibility of the authors and does not necessarily represent the official views of the National Cancer Institute or the National Institutes of Health. Additional support was provided by UCLA Clinical and Translational Sciences Institute Grant No. UL1TR000124, the Beckman Coulter Foundation, the Jean Perkins Foundation, the Steven C. Gordon Family Foundation, and the Nancy E. Barry and Letitia P. Rees Foundation.
Department of Urology, David Geffen School of Medicine at UCLA, 10945 LeConte Avenue, PVUB Suite 3361, Los Angeles, CA 90095, USA
* Corresponding author.
E-mail address: lmarks@mednet.ucla.edu

urologic.theclinics.com

INTRODUCTION

For nearly a century, digital rectal examination was the only tool available to aid in tissue sampling for diagnosis of prostate cancer (CaP).[1] With the advent of ultrasonography (US) in the 1980s, physicians had a new modality for directing biopsy needles in real time. Originally developed by Stamey, the US-guided, transrectal sextant method became widely adopted.[2] Since that time, additional samples are taken (usually totaling 12) and local anesthesia has been added, but otherwise the random, systematic procedure of the 1980s has remained largely unchanged. Saturation biopsy has been advocated but may increase detection of insignificant cancers, and it typically requires general anesthesia.

Thus, CaP is the only important solid malignancy diagnosed by blind biopsy of the organ (ie, without tumor visualization). Some 50% of cancers detected by this method may not be of clinical significance.[3] In addition, systematic biopsies are poor at sampling lesions in the anterior, midline, and apex of the prostate. This situation can lead to underdiagnosis of important lesions in these regions. Further, almost one-third of currently detected cancers are reclassified from original biopsy Gleason score to a higher score on final pathology.[4]

Groundwork for a change in this schema was established with the observation that some CaP lesions could be visualized with magnetic resonance imaging (MRI).[5] As MRI usage became widely disseminated, and as the technology improved, the value of MRI to diagnose (and stage) CaP became increasingly apparent. The advent of MRI coincided with decreasing volume of CaP at diagnosis.[6] In an earlier time, when CaP usually presented as a palpable mass, US imaging could detect many lesions. Because of early prostate-specific antigen (PSA) screening, most newly diagnosed CaP is nonpalpable, and US usually fails to visualize a lesion. Thus, use of MRI to identify suspicious prostate lesions fills an important void, helping to identify regions of interest and enable targeted biopsy.[7]

ADVENT OF MRI FOR DIAGNOSIS OF CAP

Among the first to show that CaP could be imaged by MRI was Hricak, in 1983.[5] Subsequent advances in magnet strength and the availability of multiparametric studies have made MRI the imaging modality of choice for diagnosis of CaP (**Fig. 1**). The established parameters of multiparametric MRI (mp-MRI) are T2-weighted images (T2WI), dynamic contrast enhancement (DCE), and diffusion-weighted imaging (DWI). As the limitations of PSA testing to diagnose CaP have become increasingly apparent, the importance of a visual representation of the tumor has become compelling. Accurate imaging of CaP and the offshoot, targeted biopsy, contain the seeds for a major change in management of the disease.

CURRENT USE OF MRI FOR DIAGNOSIS OF CAP

Either pelvic phased array or endorectal coils (ERC) may be used when performing mp-MRI of the prostate. ERC may improve definition of the prostate capsule, but does not seem critical for characterization of intraprostatic lesions. Thus,

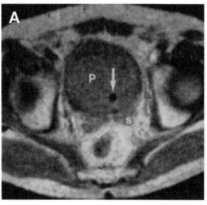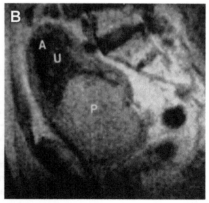

Fig. 1. Prostate MRI c. 1983.[5] These were among the first published MRI images, obtained with a 0.35-T coil. In the transverse scan (*A*), the prostate (P) is enlarged and the Foley catheter (*arrow*) in the prostatic urethra is displaced posteriorly to the left by adenomatous tissue. Seminal vesicles are seen inferior to the bladder (s). In the sagittal scan (*B*), air (A) and urine (U) level can be seen in the bladder. At the time, magnet strength was not capable of showing zonal anatomy or small cancers. (*From* Hricak H, Williams RD, Spring DB, et al. Anatomy and pathology of the male pelvis by magnetic resonance imaging. AJR Am J Roentgenol 1983;141(6):1107; with permission.)

because of patient discomfort and increased procedure time, the endorectal approach is not routinely used for diagnostic purposes. Likewise, to identify regions of interest and guide biopsy, spectroscopy adds little and is not generally used. Three-Tesla magnets provide higher signal-to-noise ratios and shorter acquisition times than 1.5 T; both have been used successfully to define cancer within the prostate.[8]

MP-MRI

mp-MRI incorporates several different imaging modalities: T2WI, DWI, and DCE to best assess potential lesions in the prostate. **Fig. 2** shows an example of CaP visualized in all 3 modalities.

T2WI produces an anatomic image based on the transverse relaxation time after magnetically aligning a tissue to an external magnetic field. T2WI provides the best tissue contrast for the detection, localization, and staging of CaP, which has shorter T2 than normal tissue. However, other processes such as inflammation and prostatic hyperplasia

can also shorten T2, and additional parameters are necessary to increase the specificity of T2WI.

DWI provides a measure of the Brownian motion of water molecules and is an essential component of mp-MRI. At body temperature, the mobility of water is primarily dependent on the molecular environment such as cell size and microstructure. DWI is a good indicator for CaP, because free motion of water is generally restricted within cancerous tissue. The slope of change of the received signal, based on the degree of diffusion weighting, is called the apparent diffusion coefficient (ADC) and creates quantitative maps of molecular mobility. By measuring the hydrodynamic environment of tissue using DWI, the specificity of CaP detection is improved compared with T2WI alone.[9] In creating the University of California at San Francisco (UCLA) score for MRI suspicion, DWI is doubly weighted, as discussed later.

DCE uses T1-shortening contrast to evaluate tumor vascularity[10] and adds value to diagnosis of suspicious lesions.[11] For this method, rapidly repeated imaging is performed during the dynamic

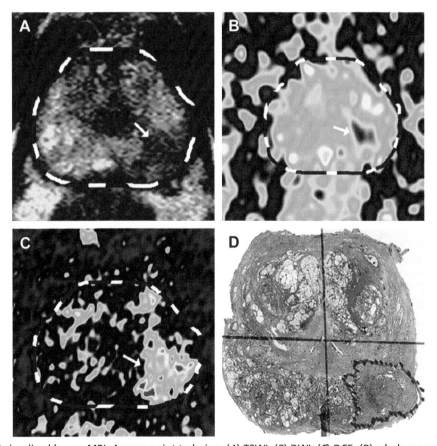

Fig. 2. CaP visualized by mp-MRI. Arrows point to lesion. (*A*) T2WI, (*B*) DWI, (*C*) DCE, (*D*) whole mount specimen obtained by radical prostatectomy, showing cancer. (*From* Natarajan S, Marks LS, Margolis DJ, et al. Clinical application of a 3D ultrasound-guided prostate biopsy system. Urol Oncol 2011;29(3):336; with permission.)

administration of intravenous contrast. Increased microvascular density and breakdown of capillary walls within tumors can lead to increased contrast arrival (washin) and dispersion (washout).

MRI-identified regions of interest are scored to help determine the likelihood of cancer in that area. Different scoring systems have been proposed, but all rely on the 3 parameters outlined earlier. The UCLA scoring system is shown in **Table 1**. Image score is determined by assigning an image-grade number (left column) to each parameter; ADC value is assigned double weighting. For example, if a region of interest was moderately dark on T2WI (ie, a grade 3), had an ADC value of 0.7 mm^2/s (ie, a grade 4), and had a DCE showing moderately abnormal enhancement (ie, a grade 3), the overall score would be (3 + 8 + 3)/4 = 3.5. The score is rounded up if the region of interest is in the peripheral zone, in this case giving

it a score of 4, and rounded down if the region is in the transition zone, in this case giving it a score of 3. The higher the score, the more likely cancer is present in the region of interest.[12] The PI-RADS (Prostate Imaging Reporting and Data System) scoring system, which is similar to the UCLA scoring system, has recently been proposed as an industry standard.[8]

IMAGE FUSION

Image fusion is the process of combining information from 2 or more images into a single image (**Fig. 3**), with the intent that the resulting image provides more information than any input image alone. Image fusion, as an aid to prostate biopsy targeting, refers to the superimposition of prostatic images (stored MRI images and real-time US images) to create a three-dimensional (3D) reconstruction, on which biopsy work is performed. The fused image result gives the operator the tumor-detecting value of MRI with the ease of use of US. Fusion devices (**Table 2**) allow the operator to electronically bring MRI to the US biopsy suite, to fuse MRI and US images into a 3D reconstruction, and under real-time US guidance, to aim the biopsy needle at suspicious regions of interest seen on MRI. Performance of the biopsy is operationally similar to that performed by urologists for several decades.

METHODS OF MRI-GUIDED BIOPSY

Three methods of MRI fusion for targeting prostate biopsy are used: direct in-bore fusion, cognitive fusion, or device fusion.

Direct MRI-guided biopsy occurs within an MRI tube (in-bore), wherein the operator compares a previously obtained MRI scan with one just acquired to guide the biopsy needle. An ERC and the prone position are used for this method of targeted biopsy (**Fig. 4**). A repeat scan is taken after needle insertion to confirm localization. In-bore fusion relies on an MRI scan before, during, and after a biopsy, which is performed in the tube itself. In-bore biopsies are usually obtained only from the region of interest seen on MRI. Systematic biopsies are usually not performed because of the extra time in-bore needed to obtain the additional cores. Because systematic biopsies are not performed, small, insignificant cancers are found less often than when the entire gland is sampled.[13] However, several significant cancers may be outside the targets, leading to a concern of missing some cancers when only the MRI target is sampled.[12]

Cognitive fusion relies on a US operator's ability to guide a biopsy needle based on an impression

Table 1			
UCLA scoring system for assigning level of suspicion to regions of interest found in the prostate on mp-MRI[a,b]			
Image Grade	T2WI	ADC (mm^2/s)	DCE
1	Normal	>1.2 × 10^{-3}	Normal
2	Faint decreased signal	1.0–1.2 × 10^{-3}	Mildly abnormal enhancement
3	Moderately dark nodule	0.8–1.0 × 10^{-3}	Moderately abnormal enhancement
4	Intensely dark nodule	0.6–0.8 × 10^{-3}	Highly abnormal enhancement
5	Dark nodule with mass effect	<0.6 × 10^{-3}	Profoundly abnormal enhancement

[a] The higher the score, the greater the level of suspicion. Regions of interest with scores of 1 and 2 are no more likely to contain cancer than normal tissue and are not usually targeted. A score of 5 indicates cancer in most cases.

[b] Although both the ESUR PI-RADS and UCLA reporting systems are standardized, there are two main differences: (1) ESUR PI-RADS uses qualitative evaluation of diffusion imaging, whereas the UCLA system uses the quantitative ADC based on a series of cases all using the same scanner platform and pulse sequence parameters, and (2) ESUR PI-RADS weights the T2 appearance, diffusion, and perfusion equally, whereas the UCLA reporting system weights diffusion twice as much as the other two.

From Sonn GA, Natarajan S, Margolis DJ, et al. Targeted biopsy in the detection of prostate cancer using an office based magnetic resonance ultrasound fusion device. J Urol 2013;189(1):87; with permission.

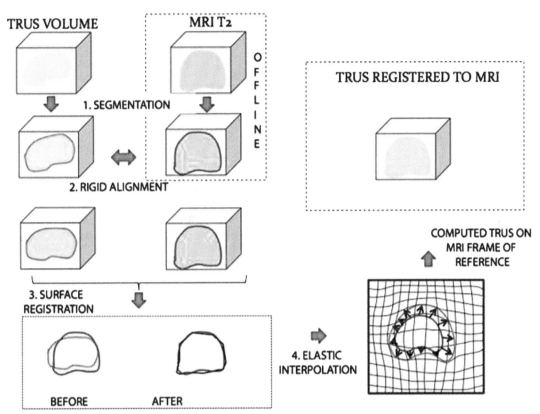

Fig. 3. Process of MRI-US fusion. MR and TRUS images are outlined or segmented (1) and then rigidly aligned (2). Fusion then proceeds involving a surface registration (3), and elastic (nonrigid) interpolation (4). The registered, or superimposed, images are produced on a monitor, where targeted biopsy is performed. The target is derived from the MRI; the biopsy aiming is via real-time US. (*From* Natarajan S, Marks LS, Margolis DJ, et al. Clinical application of a 3D ultrasound-guided prostate biopsy system. Urol Oncol 2011;29(3):338; with permission.)

gleaned from a two-dimensional (2D) MRI image. Cognitive fusion requires an experienced ultrasonographer, but otherwise is a relatively fast procedure and requires no special training or instrumentation. However, cognitive fusion does not permit quantification of targeting accuracy and is subject to interpretation of the anatomy by the operator. In a recent study from Europe,[14] the tumor detection rate of cognitive fusion was similar to that obtained by device fusion, and both were better than blind, systematic sampling. The use of cognitive fusion in biopsy site tracking, as for men undergoing active surveillance, has not been evaluated.

Device fusion uses a 3D rendering apparatus, which allows a previously acquired MRI scan to be superimposed on real-time US images, forming a digital reconstruction on a computer monitor. This digital overlay of an MRI image onto US allows the operator to obtain both systematic and targeted biopsies; in addition, biopsy sites are recorded for later repeat targeting, if necessary, as during active surveillance. An online video explaining the procedure and rationale

behind targeted prostate biopsy using MRI-US fusion has been made available (YouTube: *UCLA Biopsy*). Five fusion devices have been approved by the US Food and Drug Administration (FDA) (see **Table 2**).

MRI-US FUSION DEVICES

Image fusion for prostate biopsy (MRI-US) was first described in 2002 by radiation therapists, who used it to obtain tissue from 2 men with increasing PSA levels after treatment of CaP.[15] However, it was the work of Bax and colleagues[16] at Robarts Research Institute in Canada and that from the National Cancer Institute (NCI)-Philips collaboration at the National Institutes of Health[17] that gave rise to the commercial devices now available. Five instruments are approved by the FDA (see **Table 2**). This discussion focuses on Artemis (Eigen/Hitachi, Grass Valley, CA) and Uro-Nav (Invivo/Philips, Gainesville, FL), which have been extensively studied and are manufactured in the United States.

Table 2
MRI-US fusion devices approved by the FDA

Manufacturer/ Trade Name	US Image Acquisition	Biopsy Route	Tracking Mechanism	Year of FDA Approval	Comments
Philips/UroNav	Manual US sweep from base to apex	Transrectal	External magnetic field generator	2005	Prospective targeting, integrated with existing US device, freehand manipulation
Eigen/Artemis	Manual rotation along fixed axis	Transrectal	Mechanical arm with encoders	2008	Prospective targeting, stabilized TRUS probe
Koelis/ Urostation	Automatic US probe rotation	Transrectal	Real-time TRUS-TRUS registration	2010	Retrospective targeting, real-time elastic registration
Hitachi/HI-RVS (real-time virtual sonography)	Real-time biplanar TRUS	Transrectal or transperineal	External magnetic field generator	2010	Prospective targeting, integrated with existing US device
BioJet/Jetsoft/ GeoScan	Manual US sweep in sagittal	Transrectal or transperineal	Mechanical arm with encoders; uses stepper	2012	Prospective targeting, rigid registration

Abbreviations: FDA, US Food and Drug Administration; TRUS, transrectal US.
From Marks L, Young S, Natarajan S. MRI-ultrasound fusion for guidance of targeted prostate biopsy. Curr Opin Urol 2013;23(1):45; with permission.

All image fusion devices for targeted prostate biopsy are combinations of hardware and software to permit the acquisition, storage, and reconstruction of real-time US images. All use a tracking mechanism, a video processor, and a computer with monitor. Stored MR images are thus fused

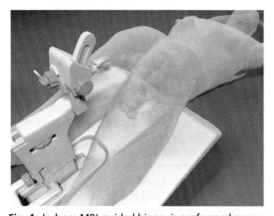

Fig. 4. In-bore MRI-guided biopsy is performed prone; the patient undergoes diagnostic MRI before biopsy; the images are then processed and delineated; the patient subsequently returns to the MRI facility for procedure, which involves fusing the diagnostic MRI with the second MRI used to guide biopsy. (*Courtesy of* Invivo, Gainesville, FL; with permission.)

or superimposed on real-time US images, allowing users to target-biopsy regions of interest identified on the MRI. In addition, 3D maps of lesion locations and biopsy sites are created and stored for future use. Movement of the patient, or movement of the prostate within the patient, affects the image registration; on-the-fly repeat registration is provided by motion-compensation software.

The Invivo/UroNav system was developed under a collaborative agreement between Philips, the parent of Invivo, and the NCI, beginning in 2006. UroNav is a modification of the PercuNav, introduced by Philips as a GPS for medical instruments a few years earlier. Tracking is performed within an electromagnetic field, created over the patient by a small generator. In 2008, Xu and colleagues[18] described the initial evaluation of a UroNav prototype, which was found to be accurate in phantom studies and in 20 patients. Since that time, more than 1000 men have undergone targeted prostate biopsy at the NCI with the UroNav device or precursor devices. In 1 recent study from that group, more than 80% of men with highly suspicious MRI lesions were found to have CaP when fusion biopsy was performed using the UroNav.[17] The UroNav system is shown in **Fig. 5.**

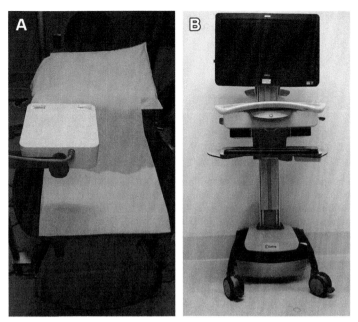

Fig. 5. UroNav fusion device. Originally developed in a collaboration between Philips and the NCI, the UroNav system uses an external magnetic field generator (*A*) for tracking the position of a biopsy needle in 3D space, which is recorded at an imaging terminal (*B*).

The Artemis device was approved by the FDA in April, 2008 and has been studied since early 2009 at UCLA.[19] The current model of the device is shown in **Fig. 6**. A developmental agreement between Eigen and the Hitachi Corporation was established in 2013. The Artemis device uses a mechanical arm for both transrectal US (TRUS) scanning and biopsy needle placement. The probe position is tracked by angle-sensing devices (encoders) within each arm joint.[16] Function of the encoders is shown in **Fig. 7**.

A summary of fusion biopsies performed with the Artemis device at UCLA Clark Urology Center is provided in **Table 3**. In the period March, 2010 to January, 2013, 501 men underwent fusion biopsy, involving nearly 8000 individual biopsy cores (5645 systematic and 2336 targeted).[12,19,20] Targeted cores were more likely to contain cancer than systematic cores (18% vs 8%), and most cancers found in targeted cores were significant ones (defined as Gleason score >6 or cancer length >4 mm).[21] Fusion biopsy in the clinic is performed under local anesthesia and is a 15-minute to 20-minute outpatient procedure. Antibiotic prophylaxis with a quinolone and a third-generation cephalosporin is used; with this regimen, among the 501 patients, only 2 episodes of sepsis have been encountered. Advantages of targeted biopsy are discussed later.

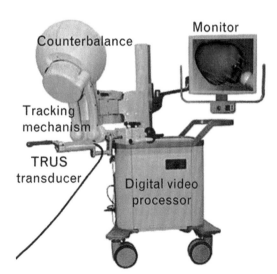

Fig. 6. Artemis fusion device. Originally developed at Robarts Research Institute in Canada, the Artemis device gained FDA approval in 2008. It is manufactured by Eigen. The Artemis device uses a mechanical arm with built-in encoders to track biopsy location. During a transrectal US scan, 2D images are digitized with a frame grabber and reconstructed into a 3D image. A model of the prostate is then generated from the 3D image; biopsy, tracking of the biopsy site, and MRI fusion are then performed on the reconstructed model. (*Courtesy of* Eigen, Grass Valley, CA; with permission.)

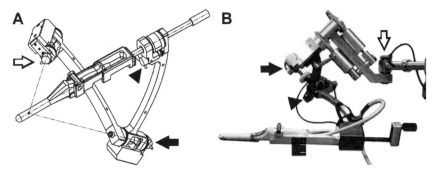

Fig. 7. Tracking arm encoders. (*A*) Prototype created at Robarts Research Institute. (*B*) Working model in current use. Arrows denote location of the 3 encoders. As the TRUS transducer and cradle are moved, encoders (*arrows*) in the tracking mechanism measure the angles between linkages, and software calculates the transducer tip position and orientation in real time. (*From* Bax J, Cool D, Gardi L, et al. Mechanically assisted 3D ultrasound guided prostate biopsy system. Med Phys 2008;35(12):5399; with permission.)

VALUE OF TARGETED BIOPSY

Targeted prostate biopsy via MRI-US fusion has proved particularly valuable in 2 clinical settings.

Previous Negative Biopsy

As seen in **Table 3**, many men seeking targeted prostate biopsy are men who have undergone previous conventional biopsy, which fails to disclose a cancer. Typically, serum PSA levels continue to increase, and anxiety brings such men to look for alternatives. In a recent report detailing experience with this group of men,[20] we found that approximately one-third of the group (36/105) harbored CaP not detected by previous conventional biopsy (**Fig. 8**). Most were significant cancers, as defined earlier. Some men had as many as 6 to 8 previous negative biopsies performed conventionally over the decade before their fusion biopsy. One had previously undergone 2 negative sets of saturation biopsies, before an anterior cancer was disclosed by MRI and diagnosed by targeted biopsy (images in the patient example below, **Fig. 9**).

Fig. 8 also shows the importance of obtaining both systematic and targeted biopsies. Significant cancer was diagnosed in 21 men by targeted biopsy alone. However, another 5 men with significant cancer (total 26) were diagnosed only by systematic biopsy and not by targeted biopsy. Thus, 5 significant cancers were found in areas of the prostate that appeared normal on MRI (ie the MRI was falsely negative in these areas). An explanation for false-negative MR images is not yet clear, but others have made similar observations.[22] An observation from several years of Artemis experience is that the biopsy map built into the Artemis software seems to provide better systematic spacing of the cores than US guidance alone.

Conventional TRUS biopsies may fail to detect CaP, especially when the tumor is located at the apical and anterior aspects of the prostate.[23,24] When MRI shows a lesion in one of these areas, targeted biopsy may be performed as usual. Saturation biopsy, regarded by many as a gold standard, increases the detection rate but also increases the numbers of insignificant cancers found.[25] Targeted biopsy may reduce the risk of delayed diagnosis for patients with significant cancer and provide increased reassurance to men whose targeted biopsy is negative.

If focal therapy becomes a treatment option, MRI-US fusion may become the method of choice

Table 3				
Summary of MRI targeted biopsy at UCLA (March, 2010–January, 2013)				
Patient Characteristics	All	Active Surveillance	Previous Negative Biopsy	Biopsy Naive
Number of patients	501	229	150	122
Median age (y)	65	65	65	65
Median PSA (ng/mL)	5.7	4.4	7.9	6
Median prostate volume (mL)	49	46	58	47
Number with cancer (n) (%)	221 (52)	148 (65)	51 (34)	64 (52)
Number with Gleason ≥7 (n) (%)	135 (27)	62 (27)	31 (21)	42 (34)

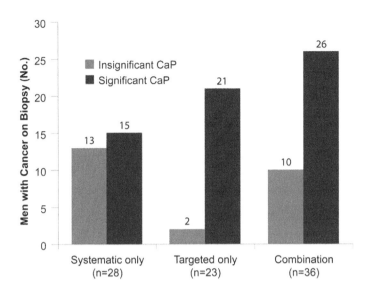

Fig. 8. Biopsy results for patients with previous negative systematic biopsies. This chart shows the number of patients diagnosed with significant cancers (*dark gray*) and insignificant cancers (*light gray*), depending on biopsy method. Clinically significant cancer was defined as Gleason greater than 6 or greater than 4 mm maximal core length.[20] Targeted biopsy detected more significant cancers and fewer insignificant cancers than systematic biopsy. Fifteen patients were diagnosed only by systematic biopsy (ie, cancer was present in areas in which the MRI showed no abnormality). The false-negative rate of MRI is not yet known. (*From* Sonn GA, Chang E, Natarajan S, et al. Value of targeted prostate biopsy using magnetic resonance-ultrasound fusion in men with prior negative biopsy and elevated prostate-specific antigen. Eur Urol 2014;65(4):809–15; with permission.)

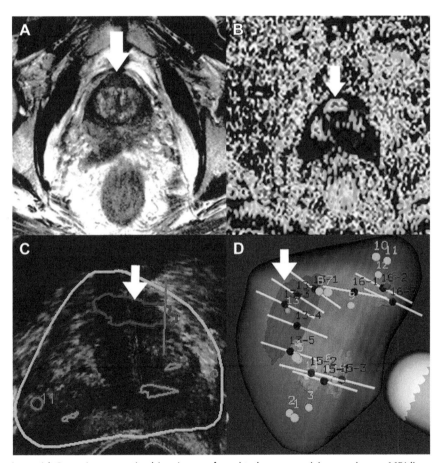

Fig. 9. A patient with 2 previous negative biopsies was found to have a suspicious region on MRI (image score = 5) and underwent targeted confirmatory biopsy via MRI-US fusion. Gleason 3 + 4 = 7 CaP was found in the anterior target. (*A*) T2-weighted MRI, (*B*) colorized ADC MRI, (*C*) US showing prostate contour with areas of suspicion outlined (large grade 5 target, *arrow*), (*D*) 3D reconstructed model of prostate showing targets and biopsy cores (*tan lines*). *Arrows* point to region of interest.

for patient selection.[26] In previous studies, perineal template mapping biopsies have been used. However, perineal mapping biopsies are more invasive, expensive, time-consuming, and morbid than fusion biopsy.[27]

PATIENT EXAMPLE: PREVIOUS NEGATIVE BIOPSY

A 70-year-old white man presented with a PSA value of 8.7 ng/mL, a prostate volume of 38.5 mL, and history of 2 previous negative conventional biopsies over the past 5 years (see **Fig. 9**). MRI showed a highly suspicious lesion at the anterior central midgland (MRI score of 5). Fusion biopsy using the Artemis device showed 3 cancerous cores from the lesion (see **Fig. 9**), including one in which the cancer occupied a length of 11 mm. Gleason score was 4 + 3 = 7. All systematic cores were negative for cancer. The patient underwent robotic-assisted radical

prostatectomy; a dominant tumor nodule of 1.9 cm was found in the anterior prostate; final pathology showed Gleason 4 + 3 = 7 CaP.

ACTIVE SURVEILLANCE

A second important use for targeted prostate biopsy is in men undergoing active surveillance for presumed low-risk CaP. This management modality continues to be underused, at least in part because of the uncertainties of conventional biopsy.[28] MRI-US fusion biopsy provides a degree of reassurance beyond that provided by conventional biopsy. Further, confirmatory biopsy via MRI-US fusion, performed after conventional biopsy had indicated a low-risk lesion, has allowed exclusion of men who would be more appropriately managed with active intervention. An example of such a case is discussed later.

Although active surveillance of CaP has proved to be safe for low-risk patients,[29] participation in

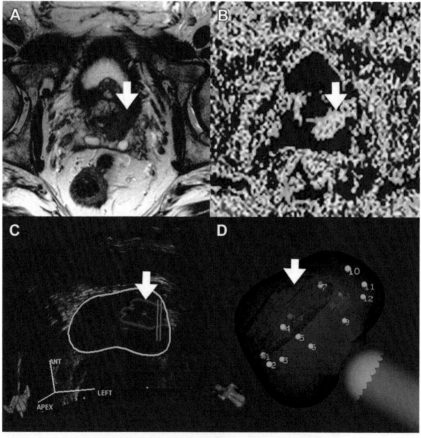

Fig. 10. mp-MRI (*A, B*) and Artemis images (*C, D*) of prostate from 64-year-old white man, who was enrolled in active surveillance from a microfocal lesion on conventional biopsy. (*A*) T2WI. (*B*) DWI. (*C*) The lesion outlined in red, superimposed on the US image of the prostate (*green circle*). (*D*) The lesion after MRI-US fusion; green dots are sites for systematic biopsy. Cancer was found only on targeted, but not systematic biopsies. Defining tumor burden in men with apparent low-risk CaP is an important use of targeted biopsy. *Arrows* point to region of interest.

such programs remains low,[30] with most recently diagnosed men electing active treatment at the outset.[31] Targeted prostate biopsy may improve patient selection for active surveillance by more accurately identifying those at lower risk. In addition, the ability to accurately return to a previous biopsy site makes fusion biopsy an ideal modality for active surveillance follow-up.

PATIENT EXAMPLE: ACTIVE SURVEILLANCE

A 64-year-old white man presented with a serum PSA level of 14.4 ng/mL and a prostate volume of 55.2 mL (**Fig. 10**). He was considered for active surveillance from an outside conventional biopsy showing 1 mm of Gleason 3 + 3 cancer. Subsequent MRI showed 2 suspicious lesions, one at the left base (MRI score of 5) and the other at the right central gland (MRI score of 3). The confirmatory biopsy was performed using the MRI fusion technique and showed 4 cores of Gleason 4 + 4 from the grade 5 lesion, with the cancer lengths measuring 3.5, 7, 10, and 15 mm. A 12-core systematic biopsy, performed at the same session, showed 2 positive cores, both with only small microfoci (3 mm of Gleason 3 + 3 = 6; 1 mm of Gleason 3 + 4 = 7). If only a systematic biopsy had been performed, this patient may have remained in active surveillance despite the presence of significant CaP. Based on the results from the MRI targeted cores, the patient underwent robotic-assisted radical prostatectomy. Final pathology showed a tumor of estimated volume of 11 cm^3 and Gleason 4 + 4 cancer.

SUMMARY

The advent of mp-MRI, which includes T2WI, DWI, and DCE, has provided a method for visualizing CaP. The MRI images may be used to guide prostate biopsy via image fusion, to enable targeted biopsy of suspicious areas within the MRI tube, or more efficiently, by MRI-US coregistration (fusion). MRI-US fusion allows prostate biopsy to be performed quickly, on an outpatient basis, using the transrectal technique familiar over the past several decades. The following conclusions represent a consensus from the initial 5 years experience, using various MRI-US fusion methods:

- Targeted biopsies are several times more sensitive for detection of CaP than nontargeted, systematic biopsies.
- Targeted biopsies detect more significant CaPs and fewer insignificant cancers than conventional biopsies.
- The false-negative rate of MRI is not yet known, but is a concern; a negative MRI

should not be used as a reason to defer biopsy.
- Two groups that will especially benefit from targeted prostate biopsy are men with low-risk lesions in active surveillance and men with increased PSA levels and previous negative conventional biopsies.

REFERENCES

1. Silletti JP, Gordon GJ, Bueno R, et al. Prostate biopsy: past, present, and future. Urology 2007; 69(3):413–6.
2. Hodge KK, McNeal JE, Terris MK, et al. Random systematic versus directed ultrasound guided transrectal core biopsies of the prostate. J Urol 1989; 142(1):71–4 [discussion: 74–5].
3. Cooperberg MR, Broering JM, Kantoff PW, et al. Contemporary trends in low risk prostate cancer: risk assessment and treatment. J Urol 2007;178(3 Pt 2):S14–9.
4. King CR, McNeal JE, Gill H, et al. Extended prostate biopsy scheme improves reliability of Gleason grading: implications for radiotherapy patients. Int J Radiat Oncol Biol Phys 2004;59(2):386–91.
5. Hricak H, Williams RD, Spring DB, et al. Anatomy and pathology of the male pelvis by magnetic resonance imaging. AJR Am J Roentgenol 1983;141(6): 1101–10.
6. Stamey TA, Caldwell M, McNeal JE, et al. The prostate specific antigen era in the United States is over for prostate cancer: what happened in the last 20 years? J Urol 2004;172(4 Pt 1):1297–301.
7. Marks L, Young S, Natarajan S. MRI-ultrasound fusion for guidance of targeted prostate biopsy. Curr Opin Urol 2013;23(1):43–50.
8. Barentsz JO, Richenberg J, Clements R, et al. ESUR prostate MR guidelines 2012. Eur Radiol 2012;22(4): 746–57.
9. Hambrock T, Somford DM, Huisman HJ, et al. Relationship between apparent diffusion coefficients at 3.0-T MR imaging and Gleason grade in peripheral zone prostate cancer. Radiology 2011; 259(2):453–61.
10. Collins DJ, Padhani AR. Dynamic magnetic resonance imaging of tumor perfusion. Approaches and biomedical challenges. IEEE Eng Med Biol Mag 2004;23(5):65–83.
11. Hara N, Okuizumi M, Koike H, et al. Dynamic contrast-enhanced magnetic resonance imaging (DCE-MRI) is a useful modality for the precise detection and staging of early prostate cancer. Prostate 2005;62(2):140–7.
12. Sonn GA, Natarajan S, Margolis DJ, et al. Targeted biopsy in the detection of prostate cancer using an office based magnetic resonance ultrasound fusion device. J Urol 2013;189(1):86–91.

13. Hoeks CM, Schouten MG, Bomers JG, et al. Three-Tesla magnetic resonance-guided prostate biopsy in men with increased prostate-specific antigen and repeated, negative, random, systematic, transrectal ultrasound biopsies: detection of clinically significant prostate cancers. Eur Urol 2012;62(5):902–9.

14. Puech P, Rouviere O, Renard-Penna R, et al. Prostate cancer diagnosis: multiparametric MR-targeted biopsy with cognitive and transrectal US-MR fusion guidance versus systematic biopsy–prospective multicenter study. Radiology 2013;268(2):461–9.

15. Kaplan I, Oldenburg NE, Meskell P, et al. Real time MRI-ultrasound image guided stereotactic prostate biopsy. Magn Reson Imaging 2002;20(3):295–9.

16. Bax J, Cool D, Gardi L, et al. Mechanically assisted 3D ultrasound guided prostate biopsy system. Med Phys 2008;35(12):5397–410.

17. Pinto PA, Chung PH, Rastinehad AR, et al. Magnetic resonance imaging/ultrasound fusion guided prostate biopsy improves cancer detection following transrectal ultrasound biopsy and correlates with multiparametric magnetic resonance imaging. J Urol 2011;186(4):1281–5.

18. Xu S, Kruecker J, Turkbey B, et al. Real-time MRI-TRUS fusion for guidance of targeted prostate biopsies. Comput Aided Surg 2008;13(5):255–64.

19. Natarajan S, Marks LS, Margolis DJ, et al. Clinical application of a 3D ultrasound-guided prostate biopsy system. Urol Oncol 2011;29(3):334–42.

20. Sonn GA, Chang E, Natarajan S, et al. Value of targeted prostate biopsy using magnetic resonance-ultrasound fusion in men with prior negative biopsy and elevated prostate-specific antigen. Eur Urol 2014;65(4):809–15.

21. Ahmed HU, Hu Y, Carter T, et al. Characterizing clinically significant prostate cancer using template prostate mapping biopsy. J Urol 2011;186(2):458–64.

22. Hadaschik BA, Kuru TH, Tulea C, et al. A novel stereotactic prostate biopsy system integrating pre-interventional magnetic resonance imaging and live ultrasound fusion. J Urol 2011;186(6):2214–20.

23. Wright JL, Ellis WJ. Improved prostate cancer detection with anterior apical prostate biopsies. Urol Oncol 2006;24(6):492–5.

24. Moussa AS, Meshref A, Schoenfield L, et al. Importance of additional "extreme" anterior apical needle biopsies in the initial detection of prostate cancer. Urology 2010;75(5):1034–9.

25. Zaytoun OM, Moussa AS, Gao T, et al. Office based transrectal saturation biopsy improves prostate cancer detection compared to extended biopsy in the repeat biopsy population. J Urol 2011;186(3):850–4.

26. Ahmed HU, Hindley RG, Dickinson L, et al. Focal therapy for localised unifocal and multifocal prostate cancer: a prospective development study. Lancet Oncol 2012;13(6):622–32.

27. Ahmed HU, Freeman A, Kirkham A, et al. Focal therapy for localized prostate cancer: a phase I/II trial. J Urol 2011;185(4):1246–54.

28. Jacobs BL, Zhang Y, Schroeck FR, et al. Use of advanced treatment technologies among men at low risk of dying from prostate cancer. JAMA 2013;309(24):2587–95.

29. Tosoian JJ, Trock BJ, Landis P, et al. Active surveillance program for prostate cancer: an update of the Johns Hopkins experience. J Clin Oncol 2011;29(16):2185–90.

30. Cooperberg MR, Broering JM, Carroll PR. Time trends and local variation in primary treatment of localized prostate cancer. J Clin Oncol 2010;28(7):1117–23.

31. Cooperberg MR, Carroll PR, Klotz L. Active surveillance for prostate cancer: progress and promise. J Clin Oncol 2011;29(27):3669–76.

Management of an Increasing Prostate-Specific Antigen Level After Negative Prostate Biopsy

Katsuto Shinohara, MD*, Hao Nguyen, MD,
Selma Masic, MD

KEYWORDS

- Repeat prostate biopsy • Transrectal ultrasonography • PCA3 • Anterior cancer
- Transperineal prostate biopsy • Multiparametric magnetic resonance imaging

KEY POINTS

- Percent free prostate-specific antigen (PSA), PSA velocity, PSA density, and PCA3 can suggest further risk of malignancy in patients with previous negative biopsy.
- Repeat biopsy should be directed to areas not previously sampled, such as anterior part, extreme apex and base, and midline.
- Changing the route of biopsy to a transperineal approach may improve the detection of anteriorly located cancers.
- Multiparametric magnetic resonance imaging (MRI) shows the cancer location with higher sensitivity than transrectal ultrasonography (TRUS) and should be considered before repeat biopsy.
- Newer tumor markers, field defect markers and MRI/TRUS fusion technology may improve sensitivity and specificity of detection of prostate cancer.

INTRODUCTION

Persistent increase in prostate-specific antigen (PSA) levels in patients with previous negative biopsies creates a clinical dilemma. Increase in PSA levels is nonspecific and can be associated with benign causes, such as benign prostatic hyperplasia, infection, inflammation, infarction, mechanical stimulation, and so forth. Despite its vague implications, urologists are compelled to evaluate increasing PSA levels to avoid missing a diagnosis of prostate cancer. With the recent increase in septicemia cases associated with prostate biopsies,[1] complications can be costly and potentially life threatening. With conventional transrectal ultrasonography (TRUS) technology, sampling errors are inevitable, and a negative biopsy does not rule out malignancy with certainty. The management of the patient with repeatedly negative prostate biopsies and clinical characteristics suggestive of cancer, such as an increased PSA level or abnormal digital rectal examination (DRE), remains a challenging problem for physicians and patients. The current TRUS-guided prostate biopsy technique may be associated with some discomfort and pain. Further, potential complications associated with biopsies are not negligible. Which findings necessitate repeat biopsy and when repeat biopsies should be recommended is difficult to determine. With low certainty of finding a high-risk cancer on repeat biopsy, the benefits of determining a diagnosis must be weighed against the risks of subjecting patients to rebiopsy-related morbidities.

Funding Sources: Dr K. Shinohara: Nihon Mediphysics, ProceptBioRobotics; Dr H. Nguyen: None; Dr S. Masic: None.
Conflict of Interest: None.
Department of Urology, University of California, San Francisco, 1600 Divisadero Street A-634, San Francisco, CA 94143-1695, USA
* Corresponding author.
E-mail address: kshinohara@urology.ucsf.edu

RISK OF FALSE-NEGATIVE RESULTS WITH PROSTATE BIOPSY

Repeat prostate biopsies detect cancer in 16% to 41% of cases in which the initial biopsy was negative.[2] At the University of California at San Francisco (UCSF), Shinohara and colleagues attempted to identify predictors of positive biopsy to avoid unnecessary biopsy procedures in patients at low risk for malignancy by studying 325 men with a history of 2 or more negative biopsies. The mean age of this patient population was 61 years, with a mean serum PSA level of 13.8. The repeat positive biopsy rate in these patients was 38%. The percentage of patients with a positive biopsy decreased as the number of previous negative biopsies increased: 40% in patients with 2 or 3 previous negative biopsies, 36% in patients with 4 or 5 previous negative biopsies, and 17% in patients with 6 previous negative biopsies. Using a Cox proportional hazards model, predictors of positive biopsy were identified, including higher serum PSA level, increased age, hypoechoic lesions on ultrasonography, and smaller prostates. Abnormal pathology (prostatic intraepithelial neoplasia [PIN], atypical small acinar proliferation [ASAP]) on previous biopsy, abnormal DRE, and transition zone volume were not significant predictors of a positive biopsy (Shinohara K, unpublished data, 2004). Clinical data accumulation now identifies more reliable predictors for patients who need a repeat biopsy in this population. Ploussard and colleagues reported the factors associated with repeat biopsy on longitudinal follow-up among patients who had initially negative biopsy. Of 617 men followed for a mean of 19 months, 31% underwent repeat biopsy. The risk factors for repeat biopsy are high PSA levels, high PSA density (PSAD), and younger age. These investigators also reported PSA levels greater than 6 ng/mL, PSAD greater than 0.15, prostate volume less than 50 mL were associated with positive biopsy results.

PREDICTORS FOR REPEAT PROSTATE BIOPSY
High-Grade PIN and ASAP

High-grade PIN (HGPIN) is found on a varying but significant fraction of prostate biopsies (1%–25%), with most modern series having an average of 5%.[3] PIN is characterized by architecturally begin prostate acini, which are lined by cytologically atypical cells. HGPIN may be a precursor lesion to adenocarcinoma.[4,5] Previously, the discovery of HGPIN on first prostate biopsy prompted repeat prostate biopsy in 3 to 6 months. Published series of those with HGPIN who undergo repeat biopsies show a cancer detection rate of 30% to 50%. However, Lefkowitz and colleagues[6] reported that with an extended biopsy scheme showing HGPIN, repeat biopsy showed cancer in only 2.3% of cases. These investigators recommended that immediate repeat biopsy is not necessary after a 12-core biopsy showing HGPIN. Netto and Epstein[7] reported a higher incidence of cancer diagnosis in patients with initial biopsy showing widespread HGPIN. More recently, Lee and colleagues[8] reported their results of 328 men undergoing repeat prostate biopsy after the initial biopsy showed HGPIN. In their study, these investigators found that a group with multifocal or bilateral HGPIN on initial biopsy had a significantly increased hazard ratio of subsequent prostate cancer compared with the unifocal HGPIN disease group. These investigators found a 3-year cancer detection rate of 29% to 37% in the multifocal HGPIN group.

ASAP, which has also previously been termed atypical adenomatous hyperplasia or atypia, is characterized by the crowding and proliferation of small glands; however, cytologic atypia is minimal.[9] This lesion has been less well characterized than HGPIN, but ASAP alone is identified in 5% of patients undergoing needle biopsy. Iczkowski and colleagues[10] proposed further classification of this lesion into 3 categories (favoring benign, uncertain, and favoring malignant) and suggested correlation of each category with subsequent cancer detection. The association of ASAP with prostate cancer is higher than that of HGPIN. Contemporary biopsy series looking at the influence of ASAP have shown that the probability of detecting adenocarcinoma on repeat biopsy is 40% to 50%. Having both HGPIN and atypia together on the first biopsy may increase the rate of cancer detection on the second biopsy to as high as 75%.[11]

The current indications for repeat biopsy within the first year based on National Comprehensive Cancer Network (NCCN) Guideline Version 2012 include ASAP found on initial biopsy and extensive (multiple biopsy sites, ≥ 2 cores) HGPIN lesions.[12]

DRE, PSA and PSA Derivatives

Abnormal DRE or abnormal PSA values lack specificity for detecting prostate cancer, especially after the first negative biopsy, with the positive predictive value of PSA detecting clinically significant cancer ranging from 25% to 40%. A PSA level in the range between 4 and 10 most often resulted in a 60% to 70% negative biopsy rate. Prostate cancer is also detected in 17% to 27% of patients with PSA levels from 1 to 4 ng/mL.[13] Furthermore, a repeat saturation biopsy also detected about 18% to 43% of cancers missed after the first biopsy in men with increased PSA levels.[14,15] Hence, PSA and DRE alone are not ideal tools for reliably excluding cancer. In men with persistently increased PSA levels with 2 or more negative biopsies, clinicians should consider the PSA velocity (PSAV), the adequacy of the initial biopsy (number of cores and location of biopsies), PSAD, family history, age, and African American ethnicity when recommending repeat biopsy. Recent studies have shown that PSAV is a strong predictor of prostate cancer in repeat biopsy after controlling for age, presence of ASAP lesion, PSAD, and percent free PSA at time of repeat biopsy. A mean PSAV of 0.73 ng/mL/y was associated with low-grade cancer on repeat biopsy, whereas a PSAV of 5.73 ng/mL/y was associated with intermediate-grade or high-grade cancer after an initial negative biopsy.[16] Previously, Loeb and colleagues[17] reported that a PSAV greater than 0.4 ng/mL/y is associated with increased risk of Gleason 7 or higher prostate cancer at time of radical prostatectomy. For men with PSA less than 4.0 ng/mL, data suggest that PSAV of 0.35 ng/mL/y or greater is suspicious for the presence of life-threatening cancer, whereas for men with PSA 4 to 10 ng/mL, a PSAV of 0.75 ng/mL/y or greater is suspicious.[18] A recent study from the Cleveland Clinic also supported the significance of PSAV in detection of high-grade cancer among the repeat biopsy population.[19] Hence, PSAV should be considered when selecting high-risk men for repeat biopsy. In addition to suspicious lesions, including ASAP and HGPIN, PSAD and prostate volume have also been shown to be strong predictors of prostate cancer and thus could aid clinicians in optimizing repeat biopsy decisions.[14]

Percent free PSA has been studied extensively in the past.[20] The NCCN guidelines recommend repeat biopsy if percent free PSA is less than 10%.[12] However, free PSA alone still lacks high specificity for prostate cancer. Within free PSA isoforms, [2]proPSA is a main isoform associated with prostate cancer. The prostate health index (PHI) is a test approved by the US Food and Drug Administration (FDA) that calculates the risk of prostate cancer by a formula of [2]proPSA/free PSA × $\sqrt{PSA}$ and has shown better sensitivity and specificity over free PSA or PSA alone.[21,22] Scattoni and colleagues[23] evaluated the performance of PHI and PCA3 in detection of prostate cancer among 211 patients who underwent biopsy and reported that PHI was more accurate than PCA3 in detecting prostate cancer in the initial biopsy setting as well as repeat biopsy setting.

PCA3

The urine-based PCA3 (Progensa) is available and FDA approved for use in risk stratification for selecting patients for repeat biopsy, with a cutoff value of 25 (a higher score is associated with a higher probability of finding cancer on repeat biopsy).[24] PCA3 is a noncoding messenger RNA (mRNA) that is overexpressed in 95% of prostate cancer.[25] The PCA3 mRNA level is measured using reverse transcription polymerase chain reaction to amplify mRNA in a urine sample after prostate massage. The score is then calculated based on total PSA mRNA concentrations. Multiinstitutional validation of the PCA3 test showed that a median score of 20 was associated with negative repeat biopsy and a score of 48 was associated with positive repeat biopsy.[24,26] Hence, PCA3 seems to be superior to PSA alone when selecting patients for repeat biopsy and may aid urologists and patients in making repeat biopsy decisions. Wu and colleagues[27] reported on 103 patients with previous multiple negative biopsies that PCA3 with a cutoff value of 25 showed sensitivity of 67% and specificity of 64%. In that analysis, PCA3, PSAD, PSA (inverse), DRE, and TRUS were all independently predictive and were included in a multivariable nomogram. The results were significantly better than PSA alone and as sensitive and specific as PSAD. However, Roobol and colleagues[28] reported that if PCA3 was excessively high (>100), the positive predictive value of the test was only 51%. Evaluation of the Genomic Applications in Practice Prevention Working Group[29] reported that the PCA3 test does not have enough clinical evidence to recommend clinical use unless further evidence is acquired to support improved outcomes at this point.

TMPRSS2-ERG Fusion

Still in the clinical trial phase, the TMPRSS2-ERG (transmembrane protease serine 2 implicated in tumor metastasis) fusion urine test is being developed to further refine risk stratification in selecting patients for biopsy. TMPRSS2-ERG fusion is reportedly one of the earliest events in prostate cancer tumorigenesis and is detected in approximately 50% of prostate cancer.[30,31] When used in combination, the TMPRSS2-ERG fusion and PCA3 urine test can give up to 90% specificity and 80% sensitivity.[32,33] This could be an attractive tool in the future for selecting men for repeat biopsy. The Mi-Prostate Score is derived from TMPRSS2-ERG fusion combined with PSA and PCA3 results and is commercially available; however, as with PCA3, more clinical data are required before recommending widespread clinical use.

Cancer Field Defect Markers

Benign tissue surrounding cancer areas has been known to have some molecular-level alterations (field defect).[34–36] By detecting those defects in negative biopsy samples, prostates with probable undiagnosed cancer may be identifiable. DNA hypermethylation in the promoter regions of cancer-associated genes is linked to prostate cancer.[37] Stewart and colleagues[38] studied an epigenetic assay evaluating such DNA hypermethylation in 498 patients who had a previously negative biopsy and underwent repeat biopsies within 30 months. Methylation-specific polymerase chain reaction assay panel was performed on initial negative biopsy samples and correlated with the second biopsy outcomes. These investigators concluded that the negative predictive value of the epigenetic assay was 90%, and unnecessary biopsies can be reliably avoided by using the test (ConfirmMDx, MDx Health, Irvine, CA). Another study using a different field effect marker[39] showed that a 3.4-Kb mitochondrial genome deletion is found in benign tissue surrounding prostate cancer. This field defect can be used as a surrogate for prostate cancer in benign biopsy specimens. If the accumulated data show the field defect markers to be clinically useful, the described tests may reduce unnecessary repeat biopsy rates and be able to target suspicious areas with high predictability.

ADVANCED IMAGING
Color Doppler and Power Doppler Imaging

Color Doppler was first described in 1993 as a potential means of differentiating malignant tissue from benign growth. It interprets reflected sound as a measure of blood flow in prostatic vessels. It takes advantage of the hypervascular nature of malignant prostatic tissue to visualize vascular flow. Increased angiogenesis in prostate cancer tissue results in higher microvessel density when compared with that of benign tissue.[40] Initial studies indicated that color Doppler could be used to identify cancers such as isoechoic, hypervascular tumors, which are not visible using conventional gray-scale ultrasonography. However, the data supporting the routine use of color Doppler are not conclusive.[41–45]

Power Doppler imaging makes use of detecting and amplifying small differences between blood flow in different vessels, allowing imaging of very small tumor vessels (**Fig. 1**).[46] This modality results in a sensitivity that is 3-fold to 4-fold that of color Doppler alone.[47] Okihara and colleagues[48] reported a sensitivity of 98% and a negative predictive value of 98%, significantly higher than that of

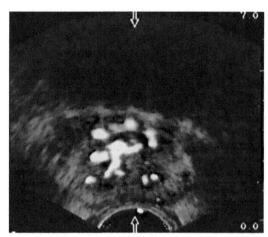

Fig. 1. A 69-year-old man with 3 previous negative biopsies. PSA level increased to 37 ng/mL. Gray-scale TRUS showed 78 cm³ unremarkable prostate. However, power Doppler imaging showed an area with significantly increased vascularity anterior to the urethra at apex. Targeted biopsy of this area showed solid Gleason grade 3 + 4 adenocarcinoma.

gray-scale ultrasonography for visualization of prostate cancer. However, in their study, the positive predictive value was 59%, equivalent to that of gray-scale ultrasonography. In addition, the patient population contained higher volume disease compared with the current PSA-screened population. TRUS studies with microbubble contrast agent enhancement have been reported. Mitterberger and colleagues[49] used contrast-enhanced Doppler imaging in 690 patients and performed both Doppler image-guided biopsies and systemic random biopsies. Targeted biopsy yielded significantly higher positive results and higher Gleason grade disease with fewer biopsy cores compared with random biopsy. Aigner and colleagues[50] used prostate biopsy under contrast-enhanced ultrasonography. Targeted biopsy yielded nearly 50% positive, whereas systematic random biopsy had only 9.3% positive. The data suggest appealing future clinical applications of ultrasound contrast agents; however, there is no FDA-approved ultrasound contrast agent available for prostate imaging in the United States.

Elastography

Elastography measures signal displacement when tissue is slightly compressed during ultrasonographic examination. This modality discriminates hard tissue unlikely to be displaced from soft surrounding tissue. Salomon and colleagues[51] compared elastography imaging with radical prostatectomy specimens in 109 patients. Elastography detected 439 lesions with sensitivity and specificity of 75.4% and 76.6%, respectively. However, when elastography was applied to targeted biopsies, 54% of random biopsies that were found to be positive did not have abnormal findings on elastography. Nelson and colleagues[52] concluded that elastography targeted biopsy could not replace systemic biopsy in the report.

Multiparametric Magnetic Resonance Imaging

Potential roles for magnetic resonance imaging (MRI) and MRI-guided biopsy (MRI-GB) in the diagnosis, staging, and management of prostate cancer have been evaluated. T2-weighted imaging improved detection of prostate cancer in men with previous negative biopsies, with a detection rate of 55%.[53] More recently, multiparametric MRI (mp-MRI), which combines T2-weighted imaging with diffusion-weighted image (DWI), dynamic contrast-enhanced (DCE) imaging, or proton magnetic resonance spectroscopy (MRS) has shown increased specificity compared with T2-weighted imaging alone.[54–56] A typical cancer is seen as an area of decreased signal intensity on T2-weighted images, restricted diffusion on DWI, rapid uptake and rapid release of contrast on DCE imaging, and increased choline+creatine/citrate ratio (**Fig. 2**, **Table 1**).

Several prospective studies have reported mp-MRI cancer detection rates between 39% and 59% in previously negative biopsy patients[57] and have found that triple combinations of multiparametric imaging modalities detect more cancers than use of only 1 or 2 of the modalities.[54] Again, most studies reported a prevalence of anteriorly located tumors.[54,58,59] MRI-GB has relatively high cancer detection rates, detects clinically significant disease, and may require fewer cores.[59,60]

REPEAT BIOPSY TECHNIQUE
TRUS-Guided Biopsy for Repeat Biopsy

When performing repeat biopsy, the standard parasagittal loci, lateral midprostate and base, anterior apex, and transition zones should be sampled. In addition, additional needle biopsies should be obtained from the site of any initial HGPIN or ASAP, as well as any suspicious lesions visualized on ultrasonography. The most common areas to be missed on initial biopsy are at the extreme apex and the base (**Fig. 3**), the midline, and the anterior regions (**Fig. 4**). Takashima and colleagues[61] carefully examined radical prostatectomy specimens from 62 T1c patients with cancer and reported that T1c cancer is densely located at the apex to midportion in the anterior half of the gland. Meng and colleagues[3] reported that adding anterior apical biopsies to the extended sextant biopsy scheme increased cancer detection, especially in patients with a normal DRE. In those undergoing repeat biopsy, additional biopsies should be directed to areas not previously sampled.

Role of Saturation Biopsy

There is no consensus on the evaluation of men with negative previous biopsies and ongoing suspicion for prostate cancer. Repeat TRUS-GB in this setting has significant limitations, because the cancer detection rate decreases with each repeat biopsy.[62]

Extensive or saturation biopsy has been recommended by some investigators to maximize cancer

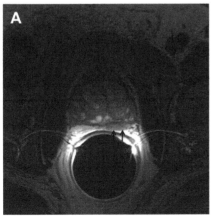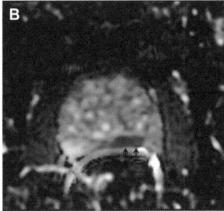

Fig. 2. (A) Typical prostate cancer on MRI T2-weighted image. Cancer is shown as an area with decreased signal intensity (*arrows*). (B) Same lesion with ADC map. Cancer site with restricted water molecule diffusion is seen as a dark area (*arrows*).

Table 1
Appearance of prostate cancer on multi-parametric MRI

	Characteristics	Cancer Appearance
T2-weighted imaging	Every tissue has its own T1 and T2 values, which can be used to generate contrast between tissues	Decreased signal intensity (dark)
DWI	Molecular diffusion of water through tissues	Restricted diffusion (bright on longer b value, dark on apparent diffusion coefficient map)
DCE imaging	Rapid T1 images are obtained after administration of contrast agent	Early enhancement and early washout of contrast
MRS	Proton spectroscopy assesses relative molecular signatures of tissues	Increased choline+creatine/citrate ratios

detection rates in patients with clinical criteria that put them at high risk for prostate cancer despite a previous benign biopsy. This type of biopsy scheme has been performed in the office using periprostatic block, intravenous sedation, or in the outpatient surgery center with general or spinal anesthetic.[63–65] Although most of the saturation biopsy protocols are performed transrectally, there are also reports of transperineal saturation

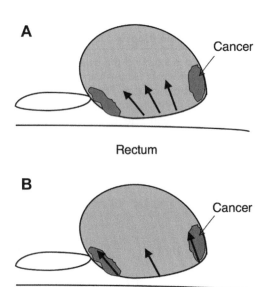

Fig. 3. (A) Example of initial biopsy (locations indicated as arrows) not taking very apex or very base tissue, missing cancer in those areas. (B) Repeat biopsy should be directed to those extreme edges where previously not sampled. (From Shinohara K, Master VA, Chi T, et al. Prostate needle biopsy techniques and interpretation. In: Scardino PT, Linehan WM, Zelefsky MJ, et al, editors. Comprehensive textbook of genitourinary oncology. Philadelphia: Lippincott Williams & Wilkins; 2011. p. 79–84; with permission.)

biopsy.[66] Generally, irrespective of anesthetic used, these saturation biopsy protocols obtain 22 to 24 cores per patient. Borboroglu and colleagues[64] found that 17 of 57 men (30%) of their cohort had adenocarcinoma identified using a 6-region, saturation biopsy pattern. Of these men, 41% had only 1 positive biopsy core; 11% of patients developed urinary retention. Stewart and colleagues[65] used a radial biopsy pattern separated by 20° to 30° and found a similar detection rate of 34% in 224 patients. The overall complication rate was 12%, which included 5% of men requiring hospitalization for hematuria. Rabets and colleagues[67] recently published a 29% overall positive biopsy rate in 116 consecutive patients who underwent a 24-core saturation biopsy regimen in the office after previous negative biopsies. This 29% to 34% rate of cancer detection is similar to repeat, extended (10-core or 12-core) prostate biopsy, which is generally accomplished with less morbidity. As extended pattern biopsy schemes become the standard of care for initial prostate biopsy, the need for secondary biopsies, by any technique, will be reduced.

Transperineal Template Prostate Biopsy for Repeat Biopsy

As stated earlier, patients with multiple negative biopsies are almost always undersampled at the anterior and apical part regions, and multiple repeat biopsy should target tissue along the anterior apical capsule. The advantage of the transperineal approach is that it allows sampling of these areas easily (Fig. 5). A transperineal approach using a perineal template also allows targeting of MRI lesions that are not seen on ultrasonography. Recently, a series of TRUS-guided transperineal template prostate biopsies showed significant apicoanterior cancer detection in patients with a normal DRE.[68] Therefore,

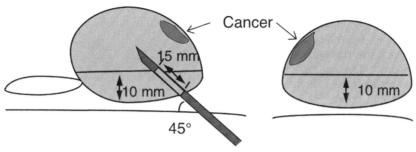

Fig. 4. Apical anterior tissue is commonly not sampled with transrectal biopsy unless the area is specifically targeted. (*From* Shinohara K, Master VA, Chi T, et al. Prostate needle biopsy techniques and interpretation. In: Scardino PT, Linehan WM, Zelefsky MJ, et al, editors. Comprehensive textbook of genitourinary oncology. Philadelphia: Lippincott Williams & Wilkins; 2011. p. 79–84; with permission.)

a transperineal approach is favored by some for secondary/repeat biopsies. Merrick and colleagues[69] performed 102 transperineal template-guided biopsies. Of those biopsies, 101 patients had previously negative biopsy and 42.2% patients were subsequently diagnosed as having prostate cancer by this approach. More strikingly, 65% of cancer cases found were Gleason score 7 or higher by transperineal biopsy. Several transperineal saturation biopsy studies have reported cancer detection rates between 20% and 68% after previous negative biopsies.[15,70,71] Walz and colleagues reported a 41% cancer detection rate with transperineal biopsy in patients with at least 2 previous negative biopsies. These investigators described a regression model that accurately predicted cancer detection at saturation biopsy 72% of the time. In their model, PSA exerted minimal predictive effect, whereas PSAD, transition zone volume, and % free PSA exerted significant effects; other studies have reported PSA doubling time and PSAV to be the only independent

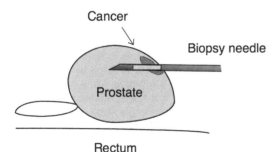

Fig. 5. With a transperineal approach, anteriorly located cancer is easily biopsied. (*From* Shinohara K, Master VA, Chi T, et al. Prostate needle biopsy techniques and interpretation. In: Scardino PT, Linehan WM, Zelefsky MJ, et al, editors. Comprehensive textbook of genitourinary oncology. Philadelphia: Lippincott Williams & Wilkins; 2011. p. 79–84; with permission.)

predictors.[72] Furthermore, Walz and colleagues found that the risk of finding cancer on transperineal saturation biopsy was highest in men with large prostates and small transition zone volumes, that is, men with large peripheral zone volumes. Bittner and colleagues reported 46.6% cancer detection in a cohort of 485 patients with previous negative TRUS-guided biopsy (TRUS-GB), 86.7% of whom harbored clinically significant disease. The most common site of cancer detection was the anterior apex, which is similar to other studies,[71] and anterolateral and posterolateral regions as well as the transition zone were also common. These investigators found that in patients with only 1 previous negative TRUS-GB result, the posterolateral region was positive as often as the anterior and apical regions. For patients with 2 or more negative previous biopsies, disease was more commonly diagnosed in the anterolateral and apical regions. These findings further support the notion that transrectal biopsies are limited in their ability to sample all anatomic regions of the prostate, especially the anterior and apical areas.

At UCSF, transperineal biopsy is performed only in patients with a high-risk clinical profile for prostate cancer who have had multiple ($\geq$2) negative biopsies. Using a transperineal approach, the direction and location of needle puncture are completely changed from the transrectal approach, allowing not only adequate sampling of the often undersampled anterior and apical prostate but also distinctly different sampling of regions usually covered in the extended sextant biopsy approach. Therefore, it may be reasonable to consider this procedure for patients with previously multiple negative biopsies and a continuous increase in PSA level or in patients with other high-risk characteristics, such as a first-degree relative with prostate cancer.

The procedure is generally performed under general or spinal anesthesia. The patient is placed in the lithotomy position, and a biplane TRUS probe is commonly used. The probe is fixed on a brachytherapy stand, and the brachytherapy template is used to guide the needle into the appropriate location.[66] The number of the cores obtained varies widely in the literature and ranges between 20 and 138 cores.[73,74] Satoh and colleagues[75] reported their procedure in detail. In their report, 4 samples were taken from each quadrant in the coronal plane at the midgland and apex, and 3 cores were obtained at each of the anterior and posterior halves, totaling 22 cores. At UCSF, the prostate gland is visualized in the transverse view and divided into 8 regions by dividing the gland into an apical half and a basal half, with 4 quadrants in each half: the right and left anterior as well as the right and left posterior gland. In each region, 4 cores are obtained (3 along the prostate capsule, 1 from the center of the quadrant), totaling 32 core samples (**Fig. 6**). Using the brachytherapy stand and template, apical coronal images are obtained. In this plane, 4 biopsy locations in each quadrant are chosen, and a needle is advanced through the preselected hole in the template. The needle is then identified in the longitudinal view and advanced until the tip reaches the prostatic capsule. Biopsy is then taken from this point in each location. After completing the 16 biopsies in this plane, the TRUS probe is advanced to the midportion of the gland. New biopsy locations on the template are chosen, and the needle is advanced to the midgland in a longitudinal view. Biopsy is taken from the midgland to the base by advancing the needle to the midgland in the longitudinal view (see **Fig. 6**B).

Biopsy of MRI Lesion

How to target suspicious lesions seen on mp-MRI has not yet been standardized. MRI-GB can be performed using a gantry adjusted to target a lesion; however, biopsy is performed outside the coil and not in a real-time fashion, and it is time consuming. Hambrock and colleagues[59] investigated MRI-GB using a technique in patients with suspicious regions on MRI and found a tumor detection rate of 59% and clinically significant disease in 93% of these patients using a median of only 4 cores. These investigators found that the detection rate was significantly higher than that of their TRUS-GB controls except in patients with PSA 20 or greater, volume greater than 65 cm^3, and PSAD greater than 0.6. Given their findings, the investigators argue that the improved sensitivity, low number of required cores needed, and sampling of areas commonly not biopsied by standard TRUS-GB make mp-MRI an appealing alternative.

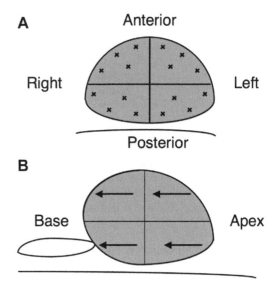

Fig. 6. (*A*) A diagram representing the location of biopsy in transverse view of the prostate. Prostate is divided in quadrants, and 4 biopsies are taken from each quadrant. (*B*) Prostate is divided in apex and base in longitudinal view. After taking 16 biopsy cores at the apex, needle is advanced to midgland, and another set of 16 cores at the base is taken. (*From* Shinohara K, Master VA, Chi T, et al. Prostate needle biopsy techniques and interpretation. In: Scardino PT, Linehan WM, Zelefsky MJ, et al, editors. Comprehensive textbook of genitourinary oncology. Philadelphia: Lippincott Williams & Wilkins; 2011. p. 79–84; with permission.)

More commonly, MRI lesions are biopsied under ultrasound guidance. Careful ultrasonographic examination of a known MRI lesion can be detected as a hypoechoic area or capsular bulging (**Fig. 7**). If TRUS shows a suspected lesion, targeted biopsy is easily performed. However, if no abnormalities are detected on ultrasonography, there are a few other ways to target the MRI lesion. Most commonly, a lesion observed on MRI is cognitively registered and geographically targeted by ultrasound guidance. If the lesion is relatively large, this approach is easy. However, if the MRI lesion is small, accurately targeting the lesion can be difficult. However, if a transperineal approach is used, the MRI lesion can be more accurately targeted by using a perineal template guide.[58]

Recently, TRUS and MRI image fusion devices were developed. These devices enable MRI lesions to be accurately targeted on the TRUS image. Sonn and colleagues[57] evaluated mp-MRI-ultrasonography fusion biopsies using the Artemis device (Eigen, Grass Valley, CA) and detected cancer in 34% of the patients and clinically significant disease in 72%. These investigators found that the degree of suspicion on MRI was the

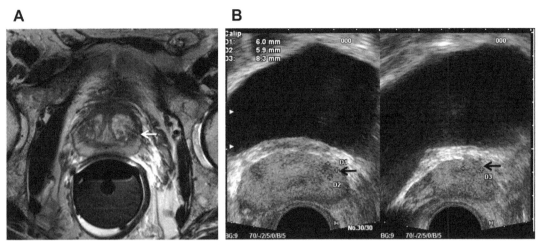

Fig. 7. A 56-year-old man with increased PSA levels. Two previous biopsies showed no evidence of cancer. (*A*) T2-weighted MRI showed a small area of decreased signal intensity in the left midgland anterior horn of the peripheral zone (*white arrow*). (*B*) Careful ultrasonography showed a small hypoechoic area (*arrows*) corresponding to the MRI lesion. Targeted biopsy showed Gleason grade 3 + 3 adenocarcinoma.

most significant predictor of significant disease. Using a different MRI-ultrasonography fusion platform (UroNav, Invivo, Gainsville, FL) (**Fig. 8**), Vourganti and colleagues[76] detected cancer in 37% of men with suspicious MRI findings. These studies reported finding more significant cancers, fewer insignificant cancers, and no detection

of high-grade cancers in men with PSAD less than 0.15 ng/mL. Similarly, Rais-Bahrami and colleagues[77] showed the usefulness of MRI-ultrasonography fusion biopsies, especially in identifying significant disease.

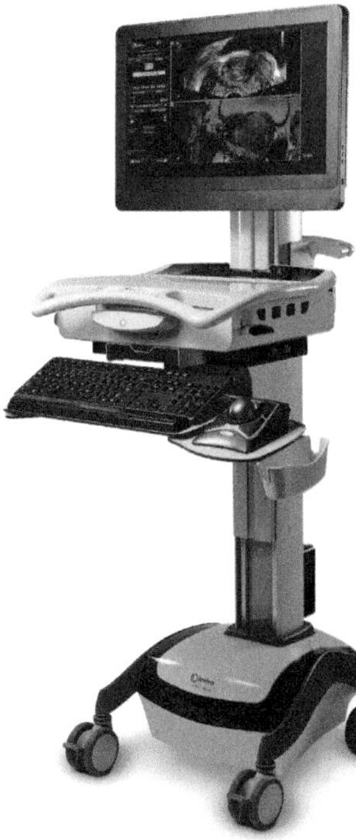

SUMMARY

Patients who have a previously negative biopsy in the setting of clinical suspicion of prostate cancer still have a high risk of harboring significant undiagnosed disease. Various markers such as PSAV, PSAD, PCA3, and newer markers may aid in repeat biopsy selection. Repeating the same biopsy procedure in such patients does not yield high cancer detection rates. More anteriorly directed transrectal or transperineal biopsies are indicated. mp-MRI can detect abnormal areas, and lesion-targeted biopsies can improve the cancer detection rate.

REFERENCES

1. Adibi M, Pearle MS, Lotan Y. Cost-effectiveness of standard vs intensive antibiotic regimens for transrectal ultrasonography (TRUS)-guided prostate biopsy prophylaxis. BJU Int 2012;110(2 Pt 2): E86–91.
2. Presti JC Jr. Prostate biopsy: how many cores are enough? Urol Oncol 2003;21(2):135–40.
3. Meng MV, Franks JH, Presti JC Jr, et al. The utility of apical anterior horn biopsies in prostate cancer detection. Urol Oncol 2003;21(5):361–5.
4. Oyasu R, Bahnson RR, Nowels K, et al. Cytological atypia in the prostate gland: frequency, distribution

Fig. 8. UroNav MRI/TRUS fusion device. (*Courtesy of* Invivo, Gainesville, FL; with permission.)

and possible relevance to carcinoma. J Urol 1986; 135(5):959–62.

5. Prange W, Erbersdobler A, Hammerer P, et al. Significance of high-grade prostatic intraepithelial neoplasia in needle biopsy specimens. Urology 2001;57(3):486–90.

6. Lefkowitz GK, Sidhu GS, Torre P, et al. Is repeat prostate biopsy for high-grade prostatic intraepithelial neoplasia necessary after routine 12-core sampling? Urology 2001;58(6):999–1003.

7. Netto GJ, Epstein JI. Widespread high-grade prostatic intraepithelial neoplasia on prostatic needle biopsy: a significant likelihood of subsequently diagnosed adenocarcinoma. Am J Surg Pathol 2006;30(9):1184–8.

8. Lee MC, Moussa AS, Yu C, et al. Multifocal high grade prostatic intraepithelial neoplasia is a risk factor for subsequent prostate cancer. J Urol 2010;184(5):1958–62.

9. Helpap BG, Bostwick DG, Montironi R. The significance of atypical adenomatous hyperplasia and prostatic intraepithelial neoplasia for the development of prostate carcinoma. An update. Virchows Arch 1995;426(5):425–34.

10. Iczkowski KA, MacLennan GT, Bostwick DG. Atypical small acinar proliferation suspicious for malignancy in prostate needle biopsies: clinical significance in 33 cases. Am J Surg Pathol 1997; 21(12):1489–95.

11. Alsikafi NF, Brendler CB, Gerber GS, et al. High-grade prostatic intraepithelial neoplasia with adjacent atypia is associated with a higher incidence of cancer on subsequent needle biopsy than high-grade prostatic intraepithelial neoplasia alone. Urology 2001;57(2):296–300.

12. NCCN Clinical Practice Guidelines in Oncology, Prostate Cancer Early Detection, Version 2.2012. 2012. Available at: http://www.nccn.org/professionals/physician_gls/pdf/prostate_detection.pdf. Accessed October 30, 2013.

13. Thompson IM, Pauler DK, Goodman PJ, et al. Prevalence of prostate cancer among men with a prostate-specific antigen level < or =4.0 ng per milliliter. N Engl J Med 2004;350(22):2239–46.

14. Campos-Fernandes JL, Bastien L, Nicolaiew N, et al. Prostate cancer detection rate in patients with repeated extended 21-sample needle biopsy. Eur Urol 2009;55(3):600–6.

15. Walz J, Graefen M, Chun FK, et al. High incidence of prostate cancer detected by saturation biopsy after previous negative biopsy series. Eur Urol 2006;50(3):498–505.

16. Elshafei A, Li YH, Hatem A, et al. The utility of PSA velocity in prediction of prostate cancer and high grade cancer after an initially negative prostate biopsy. Prostate 2013. [Epub ahead of print].

17. Loeb S, Roehl KA, Helfand BT, et al. Can prostate specific antigen velocity thresholds decrease insignificant prostate cancer detection? J Urol 2010;183(1):112–6.

18. Carter HB, Ferrucci L, Kettermann A, et al. Detection of life-threatening prostate cancer with prostate-specific antigen velocity during a window of curability. J Natl Cancer Inst 2006;98(21):1521–7.

19. Elshafei A, Li YH, Hatem A, et al. The utility of PSA velocity in prediction of prostate cancer and high grade cancer after an initially negative prostate biopsy. Prostate 2013;73(16):1796–802.

20. Catalona WJ, Partin AW, Slawin KM, et al. Use of the percentage of free prostate-specific antigen to enhance differentiation of prostate cancer from benign prostatic disease: a prospective multicenter clinical trial. JAMA 1998;279(19):1542–7.

21. Catalona WJ, Partin AW, Sanda MG, et al. A multicenter study of [-2] pro-prostate specific antigen combined with prostate specific antigen and free prostate specific antigen for prostate cancer detection in the 2.0 to 10.0 ng/ml prostate specific antigen range. J Urol 2011;185(5):1650–5.

22. Loeb S, Sokoll LJ, Broyles DL, et al. Prospective multicenter evaluation of the Beckman Coulter Prostate Health Index using WHO calibration. J Urol 2013;189(5):1702–6.

23. Scattoni V, Lazzeri M, Lughezzani G, et al. Head-to-head comparison of prostate health index and urinary PCA3 for predicting cancer at initial or repeat biopsy. J Urol 2013;190(2):496–501.

24. Auprich M, Haese A, Walz J, et al. External validation of urinary PCA3-based nomograms to individually predict prostate biopsy outcome. Eur Urol 2010;58(5):727–32.

25. Bussemakers MJ, van Bokhoven A, Verhaegh GW, et al. DD3: a new prostate-specific gene, highly overexpressed in prostate cancer. Cancer Res 1999;59(23):5975–9.

26. Marks LS, Fradet Y, Deras IL, et al. PCA3 molecular urine assay for prostate cancer in men undergoing repeat biopsy. Urology 2007;69(3):532–5.

27. Wu AK, Reese AC, Cooperberg MR, et al. Utility of PCA3 in patients undergoing repeat biopsy for prostate cancer. Prostate Cancer Prostatic Dis 2012;15(1):100–5.

28. Roobol MJ, Schroder FH, van Leenders GL, et al. Performance of prostate cancer antigen 3 (PCA3) and prostate-specific antigen in Prescreened men: reproducibility and detection characteristics for prostate cancer patients with high PCA3 scores (>/= 100). Eur Urol 2010;58(6):893–9.

29. Evaluation of Genomic Applications in Practice and Prevention (EGAPP) Working Group. Recommendations from the EGAPP Working Group: does PCA3 testing for the diagnosis and management

of prostate cancer improve patient health outcomes? Genet Med 2013. [Epub ahead of print].

30. Tomlins SA, Rhodes DR, Perner S, et al. Recurrent fusion of TMPRSS2 and ETS transcription factor genes in prostate cancer. Science 2005; 310(5748):644–8.

31. Mosquera JM, Mehra R, Regan MM, et al. Prevalence of TMPRSS2-ERG fusion prostate cancer among men undergoing prostate biopsy in the United States. Clin Cancer Res 2009;15(14): 4706–11.

32. Hessels D, Smit FP, Verhaegh GW, et al. Detection of TMPRSS2-ERG fusion transcripts and prostate cancer antigen 3 in urinary sediments may improve diagnosis of prostate cancer. Clin Cancer Res 2007;13(17):5103–8.

33. Salami SS, Schmidt F, Laxman B, et al. Combining urinary detection of TMPRSS2: ERG and PCA3 with serum PSA to predict diagnosis of prostate cancer. Urol Oncol 2013;31(5):566–71.

34. Maekita T, Nakazawa K, Mihara M, et al. High levels of aberrant DNA methylation in Helicobacter pylori-infected gastric mucosae and its possible association with gastric cancer risk. Clin Cancer Res 2006; 12(3 Pt 1):989–95.

35. Takahashi T, Habuchi T, Kakehi Y, et al. Clonal and chronological genetic analysis of multifocal cancers of the bladder and upper urinary tract. Cancer Res 1998;58(24):5835–41.

36. Kamiyama H, Suzuki K, Maeda T, et al. DNA demethylation in normal colon tissue predicts predisposition to multiple cancers. Oncogene 2012;31(48): 5029–37.

37. Yang B, Bhusari S, Kueck J, et al. Methylation profiling defines an extensive field defect in histologically normal prostate tissues associated with prostate cancer. Neoplasia 2013;15(4):399–408.

38. Stewart GD, Van Neste L, Delvenne P, et al. Clinical utility of an epigenetic assay to detect occult prostate cancer in histopathologically negative biopsies: results of the MATLOC study. J Urol 2013; 189(3):1110–6.

39. Parr RL, Mills J, Harbottle A, et al. Mitochondria, prostate cancer, and biopsy sampling error. Discov Med 2013;15(83):213–20.

40. Bigler SA, Deering RE, Brawer MK. Comparison of microscopic vascularity in benign and malignant prostate tissue. Hum Pathol 1993;24(2):220–6.

41. Ismail M, Petersen RO, Alexander AA, et al. Color Doppler imaging in predicting the biologic behavior of prostate cancer: correlation with disease-free survival. Urology 1997;50(6):906–12.

42. Arger PH, Malkowicz SB, VanArsdalen KN, et al. Color and power Doppler sonography in the diagnosis of prostate cancer: comparison between vascular density and total vascularity. J Ultrasound Med 2004;23(5):623–30.

43. Okihara K, Watanabe H, Kojima M. Kinetic study of tumor blood flow in prostatic cancer using power Doppler imaging. Ultrasound Med Biol 1999; 25(1):89–94.

44. Kravchick S, Cytron S, Peled R, et al. Colour Doppler ultrasonography for detecting perineural invasion (PNI) and the value of PNI in predicting final pathological stage: a prospective study of men with clinically localized prostate cancer. BJU Int 2003;92(1):28–31.

45. Cheng S, Rifkin MD. Color Doppler imaging of the prostate: important adjunct to endorectal ultrasound of the prostate in the diagnosis of prostate cancer. Ultrasound Q 2001;17(3):185–9.

46. Sakarya ME, Arslan H, Unal O, et al. The role of power Doppler ultrasonography in the diagnosis of prostate cancer: a preliminary study. Br J Urol 1998;82(3):386–8.

47. Rubin JM, Bude RO, Carson PL, et al. Power Doppler US: a potentially useful alternative to mean frequency-based color Doppler US. Radiology 1994;190(3):853–6.

48. Okihara K, Kojima M, Nakanouchi T, et al. Transrectal power Doppler imaging in the detection of prostate cancer. BJU Int 2000;85(9):1053–7.

49. Mitterberger M, Christian G, Pinggera GM, et al. Gray scale and color Doppler sonography with extended field of view technique for the diagnostic evaluation of anterior urethral strictures. J Urol 2007;177(3):992–6 [discussion: 997].

50. Aigner F, Pallwein L, Mitterberger M, et al. Contrast-enhanced ultrasonography using cadence-contrast pulse sequencing technology for targeted biopsy of the prostate. BJU Int 2009;103(4):458–63.

51. Salomon G, Kollerman J, Thederan I, et al. Evaluation of prostate cancer detection with ultrasound real-time elastography: a comparison with step section pathological analysis after radical prostatectomy. Eur Urol 2008;54(6):1354–62.

52. Nelson ED, Slotoroff CB, Gomella LG, et al. Targeted biopsy of the prostate: the impact of color Doppler imaging and elastography on prostate cancer detection and Gleason score. Urology 2007;70(6):1136–40.

53. Anastasiadis AG, Lichy MP, Nagele U, et al. MRI-guided biopsy of the prostate increases diagnostic performance in men with elevated or increasing PSA levels after previous negative TRUS biopsies. Eur Urol 2006;50(4):738–48 [discussion: 748–9].

54. Franiel T, Stephan C, Erbersdobler A, et al. Areas suspicious for prostate cancer: MR-guided biopsy in patients with at least one transrectal US-guided biopsy with a negative finding–multiparametric MR imaging for detection and biopsy planning. Radiology 2011;259(1):162–72.

55. Beyersdorff D, Taupitz M, Winkelmann B, et al. Patients with a history of elevated prostate-specific

antigen levels and negative transrectal US-guided quadrant or sextant biopsy results: value of MR imaging. Radiology 2002;224(3):701–6.

56. Puech P, Potiron E, Lemaitre L, et al. Dynamic contrast-enhanced-magnetic resonance imaging evaluation of intraprostatic prostate cancer: correlation with radical prostatectomy specimens. Urology 2009;74(5):1094–9.

57. Sonn GA, Chang E, Natarajan S, et al. Value of Targeted Prostate Biopsy Using Magnetic Resonance-Ultrasound Fusion in Men with Prior Negative Biopsy and Elevated Prostate-specific Antigen. Eur Urol 2013. [Epub ahead of print].

58. Abd-Alazeez M, Ahmed HU, Arya M, et al. The accuracy of multiparametric MRI in men with negative biopsy and elevated PSA level-Can it rule out clinically significant prostate cancer? Urol Oncol 2013. [Epub ahead of print].

59. Hambrock T, Somford DM, Hoeks C, et al. Magnetic resonance imaging guided prostate biopsy in men with repeat negative biopsies and increased prostate specific antigen. J Urol 2010;183(2):520–7.

60. Chiang IN, Chang SJ, Pu YS, et al. Major complications and associated risk factors of transrectal ultrasound guided prostate needle biopsy: a retrospective study of 1875 cases in taiwan. J Formos Med Assoc 2007;106(11):929–34.

61. Takashima R, Egawa S, Kuwao S, et al. Anterior distribution of Stage T1c nonpalpable tumors in radical prostatectomy specimens. Urology 2002; 59(5):692–7.

62. Roehl KA, Antenor JA, Catalona WJ. Serial biopsy results in prostate cancer screening study. J Urol 2002;167(6):2435–9.

63. Jones JS, Oder M, Zippe CD. Saturation prostate biopsy with periprostatic block can be performed in office. J Urol 2002;168(5):2108–10.

64. Borboroglu PG, Comer SW, Riffenburgh RH, et al. Extensive repeat transrectal ultrasound guided prostate biopsy in patients with previous benign sextant biopsies. J Urol 2000;163(1):158–62.

65. Stewart CS, Leibovich BC, Weaver AL, et al. Prostate cancer diagnosis using a saturation needle biopsy technique after previous negative sextant biopsies. J Urol 2001;166(1):86–91 [discussion: 91–2].

66. Bott SR, Henderson A, McLarty E, et al. A brachytherapy template approach to standardize saturation prostatic biopsy. BJU Int 2004;93(4):629–30.

67. Rabets JC, Jones JS, Patel A, et al. Prostate cancer detection with office based saturation biopsy in a repeat biopsy population. J Urol 2004;172(1): 94–7.

68. Kawakami S, Kihara K, Fujii Y, et al. Transrectal ultrasound-guided transperineal 14-core systematic biopsy detects apico-anterior cancer foci of T1c prostate cancer. Int J Urol 2004;11(8):613–8.

69. Merrick GS, Gutman S, Andreini H, et al. Prostate cancer distribution in patients diagnosed by transperineal template-guided saturation biopsy. Eur Urol 2007;52(3):715–23.

70. Bittner N, Merrick GS, Butler WM, et al. Incidence and pathological features of prostate cancer detected on transperineal template guided mapping biopsy after negative transrectal ultrasound guided biopsy. J Urol 2013;190(2):509–14.

71. Pal RP, Elmussareh M, Chanawani M, et al. The role of a standardized 36 core template-assisted transperineal prostate biopsy technique in patients with previously negative transrectal ultrasonography-guided prostate biopsies. BJU Int 2012;109(3): 367–71.

72. Mabjeesh NJ, Lidawi G, Chen J, et al. High detection rate of significant prostate tumours in anterior zones using transperineal ultrasound-guided template saturation biopsy. BJU Int 2012;110(7):993–7.

73. Pinkstaff DM, Igel TC, Petrou SP, et al. Systematic transperineal ultrasound-guided template biopsy of the prostate: three-year experience. Urology 2005;65(4):735–9.

74. Barzell WE, Melamed MR. Appropriate patient selection in the focal treatment of prostate cancer: the role of transperineal 3-dimensional pathologic mapping of the prostate–a 4-year experience. Urology 2007;70(Suppl 6):27–35.

75. Satoh T, Matsumoto K, Fujita T, et al. Cancer core distribution in patients diagnosed by extended transperineal prostate biopsy. Urology 2005;66(1): 114–8.

76. Vourganti S, Rastinehad A, Yerram NK, et al. Multiparametric magnetic resonance imaging and ultrasound fusion biopsy detect prostate cancer in patients with prior negative transrectal ultrasound biopsies. J Urol 2012;188(6):2152–7.

77. Rais-Bahrami S, Siddiqui MM, Turkbey B, et al. Utility of multiparametric magnetic resonance imaging suspicion levels for detecting prostate cancer. J Urol 2013;190(5):1721–7.

When is Prostate Cancer Really Cancer?

David M. Berman, MD, PhD[a], Jonathan I. Epstein, MD[b],*

KEYWORDS

- Prostate cancer • Gleason grade • PSA screening • Low-grade cancer

KEY POINTS

- Managing low-grade prostate cancers is a significant challenge, brought on by widespread adoption of prostate-specific antigen screening.
- Physicians who diagnose this disease and discuss treatment options with patients may move toward correctly titrating management to fit low-risk patients by shifting the classification of low-risk prostate cancers into another diagnostic category, such as a benign tumor or a tumor of low malignant potential.
- This shift is problematic in a biological sense, because low-grade prostate cancers clearly fulfill well-established definitions of cancer, and it would also be problematic in a practical sense, because risk classification by Gleason grading is often inaccurate and low-grade cancers may progress to high-grade cancers.
- In the proposed system, indolent cancers currently scored as Gleason 6 out of 10 would be assigned a score of 1 out of 5.
- The more accurate risk assessment provided by the new scoring system would be the start of a discussion between patients and physicians on how best to manage a cancer that is likely harmless.

THE SCIENCE OF DIAGNOSING CANCER

The Hallmarks of Cancer

The idea that cancer can be indolent leads to the question, what is cancer? A review published in 2000 entitled *The Hallmarks of Cancer*,[1] and its more recent revision,[2] focus on a variety of properties of cancer, including the ability to grow autonomously, evade signals that would cause programmed cell death in normal cells, invade, and metastasize (**Tables 1** and **2**). The hallmarks provide a useful heuristic device for discussing cancer biology, particularly in the context of basic research. However, hallmarks are not strict criteria for diagnosing cancer. In fact, as shown in **Table 1**, many of the hallmarks are features of benign neoplasms and therefore cannot be used to define cancer. As

carefully delineated in medical textbooks[13,14] and entertainingly presented by Lazebnik,[15] cancer is a malignant neoplasm. A neoplasm (benign or malignant) is an autonomously growing clone of cells; only malignant neoplasms invade or metastasize.[15] In practice, invasion is the only feature that is both necessary and sufficient for the diagnosis of cancer (see later discussion). Aside from invasion and metastasis, the other hallmarks are found in benign neoplasms and, therefore, not defining features of malignancy (see **Table 1**).

Metastasis Is Not a Reliable Defining Feature of Cancer

Although almost all metastasizing tumors are malignant, there are malignant tumors (cancers) that

[a] Department of Pathology and Molecular Medicine, Queen's Cancer Research Institute, Queen's University, 18 Stuart Street, Botterell 329, Kingston, Ontario K7L3N6, Canada; [b] Departments of Pathology, Urology, and Oncology, The Johns Hopkins Medical Institutions, 401 North Broadway Street, Room 2242, Baltimore, MD 21231, USA
* Corresponding author. The Johns Hopkins Medical Institutions, 401 North Broadway Street, Room 2242, Baltimore, MD 21231.
E-mail address: jepstein@jhmi.edu

Urol Clin N Am 41 (2014) 339–346
http://dx.doi.org/10.1016/j.ucl.2014.01.006
0094-0143/14/$ – see front matter © 2014 Elsevier Inc. All rights reserved.

Table 1
Hallmarks of cancer in normal tissues and neoplasia

	Proliferative Signals	Evading Growth Suppressors	Immortality	Angiogenesis	Invasion	Metastasis
Normal growth and homeostasis	+	−	−	+	−	−
Benign neoplasms	+	+	+	+	−	−
Cancers	+	+	+	+	+	+/−

almost never metastasize. These nonmetastasizing cancers can be highly locally invasive and lethal. For example, high-grade glioma brain tumors rarely metastasize, but are rapidly and almost uniformly lethal.[16] On the other side of the aggressiveness spectrum, there are several invasive cancers that carry an exceedingly low risk of metastasis. The most salient and common example is basal cell carcinoma (BCC) of the skin. Arising in sun-exposed areas, BCC is almost never fatal and carries a minuscule risk of metastasis, estimated to be as low as 0.0028% of cases. However, it can be highly invasive locally, causing disfigurement and loss of function, especially around the eyes and scalp.[17] Therefore cancers vary in their potential to metastasize, but are defined primarily by their ability to invade.

Invasive Features Distinguish Prostatic Intraepithelial Neoplasia from Prostate Cancer

Prostate cancer commonly develops from a preinvasive precursor lesion called prostatic intraepithelial neoplasia (PIN). PIN consists of neoplastic epithelial cells within preexisting benign glands. For epithelial cancers such as prostate cancer,

invading through the basement membrane defines cancer, and low-grade (ie, Gleason ≤6) prostate cancers clearly fit this criterion. The architectural features of PIN glands are those of benign prostate acini. By contrast, cancers of Gleason score 6 have an infiltrative pattern extending irregularly into the stroma, not only between benign glands but also beyond the prostate into extraprostatic tissue (**Fig. 1**A). In contrast to carcinoma, neither PIN nor benign prostate glands ever infiltrate beyond the prostate.

The replicative process of benign prostate epithelia is quite different from that of cancer. In benign prostate, basal cells give rise to luminal secretory cells as part of a differentiation program. Prostate cancer cells, by contrast, replicate autonomously. The distinctive architectural features of low-grade prostate cancer evolve as neoplastic cells invade the basement membrane surrounding PIN glands to form new glands in the surrounding stroma. The newly formed cancer glands lack a surrounding basal cell layer.[4,5] By contrast, although not always easy to identify in diagnostic specimens, both benign glands and PIN glands are surrounded by a layer of basal cells adjacent to the basement membrane.

Table 2
Features distinguishing PIN from low-grade prostate cancer in humans

Category	Feature	Benign	PIN	Low-Grade Prostate Cancer	Reference
Architecture	Glandular profiles	Large, folded, evenly spaced	Large, folded, evenly spaced	Small, round, simple	3
	Basal cell layer	Present	Present, but attenuated	Absent	4,5
Gene expression	Intense AMACR immunoreactivity on biopsy	<21%	42%–56%	>90%	6–8
Chromosomal alteration	D8S87 loss on chromosome 8p12	Infrequent	Infrequent	20%–50%	9,10
	TMPRSS2-ERG fusion	0%	12%	39%–50%	11,12
	PTEN alteration (any)	5%	15%	31%	11

Data from Refs.[3–12]

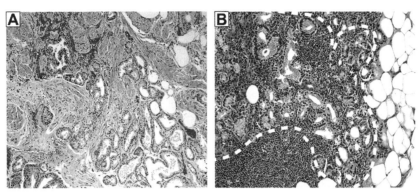

Fig. 1. Malignant properties of low-grade prostate cancer. (*A*) A locally invasive Gleason 3 + 3 = 6 cancer with pattern-3 glands invading the muscular wall of the adjacent bladder (hematoxylin-eosin, original magnification ×40). (*B*) Gleason pattern-3 cancer glands in a lymph node metastasis. Note small round glands (encircled by *dashed white line*) and adjacent lymphoid tissue (hematoxylin-eosin, original magnification ×20). Because only high-grade cancers metastasize, these low-grade cancer cells likely derive from a higher-grade precursor.

Molecular Features Distinguish Prostatic Intraepithelial Neoplasia from Prostate Cancer

The process by which noninvasive neoplastic cells acquire invasive potential is unclear. Accordingly, there are no molecular tests that accurately distinguish an invasive cancer cell from a noninvasive, in situ precursor. Nevertheless, PIN and low-grade cancers have distinctive molecular features (see **Table 1**). In addition to lacking basal cells and having smaller, simpler glandular profiles than PIN, low-grade prostate cancers express higher levels of α-methylacyl-CoA racemase (AMACR).[6–8] Higher AMACR expression seems to facilitate lipid oxidation, a favored energy source for prostate cancer cells,[18] suggesting qualitatively or quantitatively different energetic requirements for invasive growth. At the chromosomal level PIN and cancer share a variety of alterations, but PIN seems less likely to lose the microsatellite repeat D8S87 on proximal 8p,[9,10] or to show intrachromosomal rearrangements (fusions) between the TMPRSS2 and ERG genes.[11,12] The biological significance of TMPRSS2-ERG fusions is currently unclear, but they are emerging as potentially useful diagnostic features.[11,19]

By contrast, the tumor suppressor PTEN has a well-established role in the biology of prostate cancer. Genomic alterations such as gain, monosomy, and hemizygous or homozygous loss at the PTEN locus are detected twice as often in Gleason-6 prostate cancer (31%) than in PIN (15%).[11] PTEN restrains cancer growth and invasion by its inhibitory effects on downstream genes in the PI3 kinase and AKT signaling pathways. From research in animal models and clinical samples, complete inactivation of PTEN is a critical step in the formation and metastasis of prostate cancer. In humans PTEN loss is an established event in advanced cancers, whereas other kinds of PTEN alterations, including partial loss, have been recently recognized in PIN and in early prostate cancer, although their significance is unknown.[11] To better delineate the molecular basis of human prostate cancer, additional studies will need to interrogate the relationship between partial PTEN loss and activity of the downstream pathways that PTEN is responsible for restraining. In contrasting PIN and early prostate cancer, these studies may reveal more specific ways to distinguish between the two entities. In summary, although no single molecular feature perfectly distinguishes a PIN cell from a cancer cell, there are striking architectural and biological differences, and a variety of molecular features (summarized in **Table 2**) that are significantly more pronounced in cancer.

Intraductal Carcinoma of the Prostate

Special consideration is merited for a relatively rare entity, called intraductal carcinoma of the prostate (IDC-P) (reviewed by Robinson and Epstein[20]). Although not always evident on biopsy, affected cases almost always have an invasive component in addition to the IDC-P. For this reason, IDC-P is believed in most cases to represent cancerization of benign prostatic ducts by high-grade prostate cancer. Thus, IDC-P cells can reasonably be labeled cancer cells, even though they are a by-product of invasive cancer and are not invasive themselves. In the uncommon cases (∼10%) where IDC-P is not associated with infiltrating carcinoma, it represents a precursor lesion with a high likelihood of developing high-grade invasive cancer if left untreated, such that it still warrants the term IDC-P.[20]

The Race to the Basement

Two recent reviews have argued that Gleason-6 cancers are not cancer. This opinion was based on observations that Gleason-6 cancers are not only indolent but also lack certain molecular features of higher-grade cancers that can be aligned with the hallmarks of cancer and, perhaps most importantly, the claim that these cancers do not invade surrounding tissues.[21,22] Although the discussion above has dispensed with the idea that other cancer hallmarks can be used to define cancer (see earlier discussion and **Table 1**), the idea that low-grade cancers do not invade deserves extra scrutiny. Supporting evidence for this idea included the fact that low-grade prostate cancers rarely grow when transplanted into mice, and that there is less development of basement membrane around high-grade cancers than there is around low-grade cancers.[23,24] However, the ability to grow in mice is not a useful defining feature of cancer, as even high-grade and metastatic prostate cancers also often fail to grow as transplants.[25,26] It is also well established that invasive prostate cancer cells, both primary and metastatic, produce new basement membrane.[27,28] Therefore, the presence or absence of basement membrane around a cell is not a reliable indicator of invasiveness or malignancy. Of equal or greater importance, Gleason-6 cancers can be observed in extraprostatic tissue (see **Fig. 1**A). This observation indicates that these cancer cells not only escaped their original basement membrane, but invaded through benign tissue to escape the prostate. It would seem that, this evidence fulfills any logical definition of invasiveness as applied to cancer.

Which Prostate Cancer Cells Invade and Metastasize?

Lavery and Droller[22] present a somewhat more radical argument that Gleason-6 cancers do not evolve into higher-grade cancers. Instead, PIN can evolve into either a pattern-3 clone or a pattern-4 clone. In their model, pattern-3 clones give rise to a noninvasive lesion, akin to PIN. Only pattern-4 clones are invasive in this model, and they arise through a distinct morphologic and molecular pathway. As supporting evidence, the investigators cited studies of men with metastases after prostatectomy in which multiple cancers were found in the prostate, but only a single clone from each cancer gave rise to metastases.[29,30] The investigators illustrate an interesting question regarding prostate cancer clones that give rise to metastases: If Gleason 3 + 3 = 6 cancers cannot metastasize, then how do Gleason 3 + 4 = 7 cancers metastasize?

The two alternatives are that Gleason 3 + 3 = 6 cancers can evolve into Gleason 3 + 4 = 7 cancers, or that Gleason pattern 4 evolves independently. Both pathways are possible. A recent genomic study found that patterns 3 and 4 in Gleason 3 + 4 = 7 cancers are essentially clonal.[31] This conclusion agrees with common observations in prostate pathology. In examining prostate cancer metastases, one can find pattern-3 glands admixed with higher-grade glands (see **Fig. 1**B).[32] Because only cancers with pattern 4 or 5 can metastasize, this observation indicates that a single cancer cell can produce both low-grade and higher-grade progeny. Thus low-grade and high-grade glands are likely two differentiation states in the same pathway. Furthermore, Gleason grade is highly correlated with tumor volume[33]; the most parsimonious model would be one in which low-grade tumors evolve into high-grade tumors as they grow. However, one could also explain the data based on the increased growth rate of higher-grade carcinomas. It has also been demonstrated that high-grade carcinoma can arise de novo without going through a pathway of dedifferentiation of lower-grade cancers.[34] There are patients who have been followed for many years with cancer of Gleason score 6, who then are found to have higher-grade cancer. The unresolved issue is whether these high-grade cancers represent progression of the previously diagnosed lower-grade cancer or emergence a new tumor. It can be argued that if Gleason score 3 + 4 = 7 or 4 + 3 = 7 is cancer whereby a prognostic component of the cancer is the pattern 3, then when a tumor is pure pattern 3 (ie, Gleason score 3 + 3 = 6) why would it not still be cancer?

THE PROBLEM OF DIAGNOSING GLEASON SCORE 6 AS CANCER

Most Prostate Cancers are Not Life-Threatening

Prostate cancer is primarily a disease of older men that progresses slowly over the course of decades. These characteristics, along with its early detection via prostate-specific antigen (PSA) screening, makes it unlikely that a man diagnosed with prostate cancer of Gleason score 6 will die of or even be harmed by prostate cancer.

The Modern Gleason Scoring System

At present, the best way to assess whether a particular man's cancer poses a risk is to use a multivariable instrument, and to date the Gleason score has reliably been the most powerful variable. When accurately assessed (ie, by thorough examination of a radical prostatectomy specimen), the Gleason score is a potent predictor of metastasis and death. The Gleason system defines 5 morphologic patterns. However, recent modifications to Gleason scoring have eliminated patterns 1 and 2 from common use,[35] leaving patterns 3, 4, and 5 as the major recognized forms of prostate cancer. The Gleason score is the sum of the most prevalent and second most prevalent Gleason patterns at radical prostatectomy and the sum of the most prevalent and highest Gleason patterns on biopsy. Thus, a 3 + 4 = 7 cancer is predominantly pattern 3 but also has a pattern-4 component. Tumors containing only pattern 3 receive a Gleason Score of 3 + 3 = 6. These low-grade cancers do not metastasize,[36] and are therefore highly unlikely to cause harm. Cancers with patterns 4 and 5 are responsible for all or nearly all prostate cancer–specific morbidity and mortality.[37] These are the observations that have prompted some experts in the field to question whether low-grade Gleason-6 prostate cancer merits the label cancer.[21,22,38,39]

The Updated Gleason Scoring System Starts at 6 Out of 10

One problematic aspect of the current Gleason grading system derives from the fact that Gleason scores effectively range from 6 to 10. As previously noted,[38,40] if men with low-grade cancers are told that their Gleason grade is 6 out of a possible 10, this can lead to the misunderstanding that low-grade cancers are serious and should be treated aggressively.

Overtreatment of Prostate Cancer

Debate rages as to whether detecting and treating prostate cancer saves lives. Indeed, several recent high-profile publications argue that treatment of low-risk cancer may not.[41,42] A major contributor to this problem is that only half of the men diagnosed with prostate cancer have life-threatening cancer with Gleason grades of 7 or higher, yet 90% of patients receive radical treatment.[43] More startling, perhaps, is that treatment rates are just as high for the men with the lowest-risk cancers as it is for those with higher-risk cancers.[43] Thus, because almost half of the men diagnosed with prostate cancer have low-risk disease, almost half of the men treated for prostate cancer are probably treated unnecessarily. Experts are working to more selectively target treatment to those most likely to benefit. Selective treatment will require that men with indolent cancers forgo or delay treatment. However, there are several challenges in reassuring a man that his cancer

does not need definitive treatment, including anxiety associated with the diagnosis of cancer and the vagaries of Gleason grading on small biopsies at the time of diagnosis. These challenges, discussed next, have motivated several experts to ask whether low-grade prostate cancer should be labeled as cancer.

THE PROBLEMS OF NOT DIAGNOSING GLEASON SCORE 6 AS CANCER

Nickel and Speakman[39] cogently argued that Gleason-6 prostate cancers are essentially harmless, but should be considered as potential precursors of more harmful cancers. Because these cancers neither metastasize nor kill, the investigators questioned whether it might be appropriate to call Gleason-6 cancers "benign disease." The review stands as a useful rhetorical exercise in that it aims to break the knee-jerk reflex of treating every cancer that is diagnosed. Similarly, Esserman and colleagues[44] more recently proposed to reclassify cancers without metastatic potential as IDLE (indolent lesions of epithelial origin) conditions. These investigators bring up the analogy of using the term "papillary urothelial neoplasm of low malignant potential (PUNLMP)" in the bladder. One of the authors of the current article (J.I.E.) was the lead author on the article proposing the term PUNLMP, such that the current authors have no intrinsic disagreement with avoiding the "cancer" word when appropriate, so that patients are not unduly worried and not overtreated. The critical difference between the issue of PUNLMP on transurethral resection of the bladder and Gleason 3 + 3 = 6 on needle biopsy is sampling. With PUNLMP, the entire lesion is typically well visualized and removed in toto for histologic examination. With prostate biopsy showing Gleason score 3 + 3 = 6, there is an approximately 25% risk of there being higher-grade unsampled cancer. Assume we have a patient with a 12-core biopsy with 8 cores extensively involved by cancer of Gleason score 6, with a serum PSA of greater than 10 ng/mL and a palpable lesion. Given that this patient has a high risk of "upgrade" between biopsy and prostatectomy, would we call this an IDLE tumor, not requiring therapy? If one could virtually guarantee that a Gleason score 6 on biopsy was representative of the entire tumor, there could be a more persuasive case to changing its designation. As opposed to the situation with PUNLMP, there still remains the issue that even if we could be sure there was only cancer present of Gleason score 6, there is the potential for progression if the cancer is not removed.

Of perhaps equal importance is the need to be scientifically and logically consistent when defining cancer.[45] PUNLMP does not have the morphologic features of cancer, either cytologically or architecturally. Gleason score 3 + 3 = 6 cancer, in contrast, meets scientific, morphologic, and pathologic criteria for cancer, as defined across a variety of organ sites.

Risk Associated with Downgrading Gleason 6 to a Benign Disease

Diagnostic inaccuracy makes it dangerous to dismiss low-grade cancers as benign. Between 25% and 50% of prostate needle biopsies diagnosed as low grade (Gleason ≤6) come from men with higher-grade disease.[46–48] This phenomenon, called "upgrading" between biopsy and prostatectomy, means that men diagnosed with indolent prostate cancers often have higher-grade, higher-risk cancers missed on biopsy because of sampling error or difficulty interpreting small lesions on biopsy. In addition, as discussed earlier, there is experimental and observational data that some Gleason-6 cancers can progress to higher-grade tumors. Thus, responsible care of a man diagnosed with Gleason-6 cancer requires continued follow-up to monitor for the appearance of a potentially lethal cancer. If patients diagnosed with Gleason-6 cancer are told they do not have cancer, it is likely that a significant proportion will not be motivated to seek continued care and run the risk of developing advanced, incurable disease.

A SOLUTION THAT MATCHES THE BIOLOGY WITH THE BEHAVIOR

Prostate cancer is not the only tumor that is indolent. Non-melanoma skin cancer, like low-grade prostate carcinoma, is morphologically a carcinoma yet has a negligible risk of mortality. Patients are reassured about the typically benign clinical course of these cancers and consequently are not overly concerned with their diagnosis, accepting conservative treatment. Patients and physicians need to be educated about the indolent behavior of Gleason-6 tumors and alternatives to immediate treatment. To better reflect the risk of harm from prostate cancer, Pierorazio and colleagues[40] have proposed 5 prognostic categories that can be reported based on prostate biopsy (**Table 3**). For men undergoing radical prostatectomy from 2004 to 2011, these prognostic grading groups from 1 to 5 have been associated with 5-year biochemical recurrence-free survivals of 94.6%, 82.7%, 65.1%, 63.1%, and 34.5%, respectively.[40] This system retains the proven prognostic value of the Gleason system and allows continued comparison with

Table 3
New Gleason scoring system proposed by Pierorazio and colleagues (2013)

Prognostic Grade Group	Gleason Score	5-Year Recurrence-Free Survival After Prostatectomy (%)
I	2–6	95
II	3 + 4 = 7	83
III	4 + 3 = 7	65
IV	8	63
V	9–10	35

Adapted from Pierorazio PM, Walsh PC, Partin AW, et al. Prognostic Gleason grade grouping: data based on the modified Gleason scoring system. BJU Int 2013;111:759; with permission.

older literature, while emphasizing for patients and physicians that Gleason score 6 should be considered in the context of a prognostic category of 1 out of 5, not 6 out of 10. This approach will alleviate some of the fear associated with a diagnosis of Gleason score 6 "cancer" and give patients a more realistic perspective regarding their prognosis.

SUMMARY

Managing low-grade prostate cancers is a significant challenge, brought on by widespread adoption of PSA screening. Historically, as many as 90% of men with prostate cancer receive aggressive treatment, even if their cancer is classified in the lowest risk category.[43] As physicians who diagnose this disease and discuss treatment options with patients, how do we move toward correctly titrating management to fit low-risk patients? One option is to shift the classification of low-risk prostate cancers into another diagnostic category, such as a benign tumor or a tumor of low malignant potential. This shift is problematic in a biological sense, because low-grade prostate cancers clearly fulfill well-established definitions of cancer. It would also be problematic in a practical sense, because risk classification by Gleason grading is often inaccurate and because low-grade cancers may progress to high-grade cancers. Rather than a new diagnostic category, the authors favor a change in prognostic categories.[38,40] In the proposed system, indolent cancers currently scored as Gleason 6 out of 10 would be assigned a score of 1 out of 5. The more accurate risk assessment provided by the new scoring system would be the start of a discussion between patients and physicians on how best to manage a cancer that is likely harmless.

REFERENCES

1. Hanahan D, Weinberg RA. The hallmarks of cancer. Cell 2000;100:57–70.
2. Hanahan D, Weinberg RA. Hallmarks of cancer: the next generation. Cell 2011;144:646–74.
3. Egevad L. Recent trends in Gleason grading of prostate cancer: I. Pattern interpretation. Anal Quant Cytol Histol 2008;30(4):190–8.
4. Hedrick L, Epstein JI. Use of keratin 903 as an adjunct in the diagnosis of prostate carcinoma. Am J Surg Pathol 1989;13:389–96.
5. Totten RS, Heinemann MW, Hudson PB, et al. Microscopic differential diagnosis of latent carcinoma of prostate. AMA Arch Pathol 1953;55:131–41.
6. Evans AJ. Alpha-methylacyl CoA racemase (P504S): overview and potential uses in diagnostic pathology as applied to prostate needle biopsies. J Clin Pathol 2003;56:892–7.
7. Häggarth L, Hägglöf C, Jaraj SJ, et al. Diagnostic biomarkers of prostate cancer. Scand J Urol Nephrol 2011;45:60–7.
8. Wu CL, Yang XJ, Tretiakova M, et al. Analysis of alpha-methylacyl-CoA racemase (P504S) expression in high-grade prostatic intraepithelial neoplasia. Hum Pathol 2004;35:1008–13.
9. Häggman MJ, Wojno KJ, Pearsall CP, et al. Allelic loss of 8p sequences in prostatic intraepithelial neoplasia and carcinoma. Urology 1997;50:643–7.
10. Prasad MA, Trybus TM, Wojno KJ, et al. Homozygous and frequent deletion of proximal 8p sequences in human prostate cancers: identification of a potential tumor suppressor gene site. Genes Chromosomes Cancer 1998;23:255–62.
11. Bismar TA, Yoshimoto M, Vollmer RT, et al. PTEN genomic deletion is an early event associated with ERG gene rearrangements in prostate cancer. BJU Int 2011;107:477–85.
12. Mosquera JM, Perner S, Genega EM, et al. Characterization of TMPRSS2-ERG fusion high-grade prostatic intraepithelial neoplasia and potential clinical implications. Clin Cancer Res 2008;14:3380–5.
13. Cooper GM. Elements of human cancer. Boston: Jones and Bartlett Publishers; 1992.
14. Robbins SL, Kumar V. Robbins and Cotran pathologic basis of disease. Philadelphia: Saunders/Elsevier; 2010.
15. Lazebnik Y. What are the hallmarks of cancer? Nat Rev Cancer 2010;10:232–3.
16. Tran B, Rosenthal MA. Survival comparison between glioblastoma multiforme and other incurable cancers. J Clin Neurosci 2010;17:417–21.
17. Chinem VP, Miot HA. Epidemiology of basal cell carcinoma. An Bras Dermatol 2011;86:292–305.
18. Liu Y. Fatty acid oxidation is a dominant bioenergetic pathway in prostate cancer. Prostate Cancer Prostatic Dis 2006;9:230–4.
19. Salagierski M, Schalken JA. Molecular diagnosis of prostate cancer: PCA3 and TMPRSS2:ERG gene fusion. J Urol 2012;187:795–801.
20. Robinson BD, Epstein JI. Intraductal carcinoma of the prostate without invasive carcinoma on needle biopsy: emphasis on radical prostatectomy findings. J Urol 2010;184:1328–33.
21. Ahmed HU, Arya M, Freeman A, et al. Do low-grade and low-volume prostate cancers bear the hallmarks of malignancy? Lancet Oncol 2012;13:e509–17.
22. Lavery HJ, Droller MJ. Do Gleason patterns 3 and 4 prostate cancer represent separate disease states? J Urol 2012;188:1667–75.
23. Bostwick DG, Leske DA, Qian J, et al. Prostatic intraepithelial neoplasia and well differentiated adenocarcinoma maintain an intact basement membrane. Pathol Res Pract 1995;191:850–5.
24. Fuchs ME, Brawer MK, Rennels MA, et al. The relationship of basement membrane to histologic grade of human prostatic carcinoma. Mod Pathol 1989;2:105–11.
25. Carvalho FL, Simons BW, Antonarakis ES, et al. Tumorigenic potential of circulating prostate tumor cells. Oncotarget 2013;4:413–21.
26. Priolo C, Agostini M, Vena N, et al. Establishment and genomic characterization of mouse xenografts of human primary prostate tumors. Am J Pathol 2010;176:1901–13.
27. Bonkhoff H, Wernert N, Dhom G, et al. Distribution of basement membranes in primary and metastatic carcinomas of the prostate. Hum Pathol 1992;23:934–9.
28. Pföhler C, Fixemer T, Jung V, et al. In situ hybridization analysis of genes coding collagen IV alpha1 chain, laminin beta1 chain, and S-laminin in prostate tissue and prostate cancer: increased basement membrane gene expression in high-grade and metastatic lesions. Prostate 1998;36:143–50.
29. Liu W, Laitinen S, Khan S, et al. Copy number analysis indicates monoclonal origin of lethal metastatic prostate cancer. Nat Med 2009;15:559–65.
30. Mehra R, Tomlins SA, Yu J, et al. Characterization of TMPRSS2-ETS gene aberrations in androgen-independent metastatic prostate cancer. Cancer Res 2008;68:3584–90.
31. Sowalsky AG, Ye H, Bubley GJ, et al. Clonal progression of prostate cancers from Gleason grade 3 to grade 4. Cancer Res 2012;73:1050–5.
32. Cheng L, Slezak J, Bergstralh EJ, et al. Dedifferentiation in the metastatic progression of prostate carcinoma. Cancer 1999;86:657–63.
33. Merrill MM, Lane BR, Reuther AM, et al. Tumor volume does not predict for biochemical recurrence after radical prostatectomy in patients with surgical Gleason score 6 or less prostate cancer. Urology 2007;70:294–8.
34. Epstein JI, Carmichael MJ, Partin AW, et al. Small high grade adenocarcinoma of the prostate in radical prostatectomy specimens performed for

nonpalpable disease: pathogenetic and clinical implications. J Urol 1994;151:1587–92.

35. Berney DM. Low Gleason score prostatic adenocarcinomas are no longer viable entities. Histopathology 2007;50:683–90.

36. Ross HM, Kryvenko ON, Cowan JE, et al. Do adenocarcinomas of the prostate with Gleason score (GS) ≤6 have the potential to metastasize to lymph nodes? Am J Surg Pathol 2012;36:1346–52.

37. Eggener SE, Scardino PT, Walsh PC, et al. Predicting 15-year prostate cancer specific mortality after radical prostatectomy. J Urol 2011;185:869–75.

38. Carter HB, Partin AW, Walsh PC, et al. Gleason score 6 adenocarcinoma: should it be labeled as cancer? J Clin Oncol 2012;30:4294–6.

39. Nickel JC, Speakman M. Should we really consider Gleason 6 prostate cancer? BJU Int 2012;109: 645–6.

40. Pierorazio PM, Walsh PC, Partin AW, et al. Prognostic Gleason grade grouping: data based on the modified Gleason scoring system. BJU Int 2013; 111:753–60.

41. Moyer VA. Screening for prostate cancer: U.S. preventive services task force recommendation statement. Ann Intern Med 2012;157:120–34.

42. Wilt TJ, Brawer MK, Jones KM, et al. Radical prostatectomy versus observation for localized prostate cancer. N Engl J Med 2012;367:203–13.

43. Cooperberg MR, Broering JM, Carroll PR. Time trends and local variation in primary treatment of localized prostate cancer. J Clin Oncol 2010;28: 1117–23.

44. Esserman LJ, Thompson IM Jr, Reid B. Overdiagnosis and overtreatment in cancer: an opportunity for improvement. JAMA 2013;310:797–8.

45. Robey RB. Changing the terminology of cancer. JAMA 2014;311:202–3.

46. Epstein JI, Feng Z, Trock BJ, et al. Upgrading and downgrading of prostate cancer from biopsy to radical prostatectomy: incidence and predictive factors using the modified Gleason grading system and factoring in tertiary grades. Eur Urol 2012;61:1019–24.

47. Davies JD, Aghazadeh MA, Phillips S, et al. Prostate size as a predictor of Gleason score upgrading in patients with low risk prostate cancer. J Urol 2011; 186:2221–7.

48. Kvåle R, Møller B, Wahlqvist R, et al. Concordance between Gleason scores of needle biopsies and radical prostatectomy specimens: a population-based study. BJU Int 2009;103:1647–54.

Index

Note: Page numbers of article titles are in **boldface** type.

Urol Clin N Am 41 (2014) 347–351
http://dx.doi.org/10.1016/S0094-0143(14)00022-6
0094-0143/14/$ – see front matter © 2014 Elsevier Inc. All rights reserved.

urologic.theclinics.com